NECK AND ARM
PAIN

NECK AND ARM PAIN
EDITION 3

RENE CAILLIET, M.D.

Professor and Chairman Emeritus
Department of Physical Medicine and Rehabilitation
School of Medicine
University of Southern California
Los Angeles, California

Director
Rehabilitation Services
Santa Monica Hospital Medical Center
Santa Monica, California

Illustrations by R. Cailliet, M.D.

 F.A. Davis Company • Philadelphia

F. A. Davis Company
1915 Arch Street
Philadelphia, PA 19103

Other titles by Rene Cailliet from F. A. Davis Company:

Foot and Ankle Pain
Hand Pain and Impairment
Knee Pain and Disability
Low Back Pain
Scoliosis
The Shoulder in Hemiplegia
Shoulder Pain
Soft Tissue Pain and Disability

Printed in the United States of America

Last digit indicates print number: 10 9 8 7 6 5 4

Library of Congress Cataloging-in-Publication Data

Cailliet, Rene.
  Neck and arm pain/Rene Cailliet: illustrations by R. Cailliet. Ed. 3.
  Includes bibliographical references. Includes index.
  ISBN 0-8036-1610-4 (soft cover)
  1. Neck pain. 2. Brachialgia. I. Title.
  [DNLM: 1. Arm. 2. Neck. 3. Pain. 4. Shoulder. WE 805 C134n]
RC936.C26   1990
617.5′3 — dc20   90-13849

NOTE: As new scientific information becomes available through basic and clinical research, recommended treatments and drug therapies undergo changes. The author(s) and publisher have done everything possible to make this book accurate, up-to-date, and in accord with accepted standards at the time of publication. The authors, editors and publisher are not responsible for errors or omissions or for consequences from application of the book, and make no warranty, expressed or implied, in regard to the contents of the book. Any practice described in this book should be applied by the reader in accordance with professional standards of care used in regard to the unique circumstances that may apply in each situation. The reader is advised always to check product information (package inserts) for changes and new information regarding dose and contraindications before administering any drug. Caution is especially urged when using new or infrequently ordered drugs.

Preface to
Third Edition

The complaints of neck pain, or of arm pain originating from the neck, constitute a major portion of the complaints confronting the average general practitioner, physical and occupational therapist, the insurance carrier, the workman's compensation carrier, and the attorney.

As the years pass, there are continuing research efforts to ascertain the pathologic changes occurring in the tissues involved. Tissues implicated in the production of pain and impairment are continually being better identified and understood. Numerous techniques for both conservative and surgical treatment are being refined.

Newer diagnostic procedures such as computerized tomography scanning (CT), magnetic resonance imaging (MRI), evoked potential electromyography, and newer techniques of myelography and thermography, are heralding newer concepts of pathology and evoking earlier, more precise, diagnostic procedures. The patient also benefits from more precise and more effective therapeutic measures.

The legal aspects of neck injuries (whether posttraumatic as a result of vehicular accident or industrially incurred) are better documented, and proper apportionment results.

The basis for proper clinical diagnosis remains the patient's history and the physical examination. The adage that recommends reproducing the characteristic pain by appropriate position and movement is nowhere more apt than in the treatment of the cervical spine. Reproducing the precise symptom by a specific movement and/or position and knowing the anatomic significance and its impact on the appropriate nociceptive tissues, assures a proper anatomic diagnosis.

The concepts of pain—acute, recurrent, or chronic—are evolving rapidly. It is no longer sufficient merely to determine the exact tissue involved in the pain process. The mechanism of tissue injury must also be determined. The aspect leading to the progression of acute pain to chronic pain must be elicited in the early acute phase and the factors leading to chronicity must be determined and prevented.

This edition has been *completely rewritten*, not merely modified.

The functional anatomy section has been reviewed to enhance its clinical significance, with division into upper and lower cervical segments clarifying the diagnostic and pathologic differentiations. The symptomatology of each segment has been clarified. Symptoms occurring from pathology of the upper segment as compared with those from that of the lower segments have been differentiated.

The ligamentous structures have been given full discussion and are illustrated with new drawings.

The neurologic supply to the cervical spine has been given a new approach to explain the meaning of a thorough examination and the symptoms elicited in a careful history. Thorough review of a meaningful neurologic examination has been emphasized.

Occipital neuralgia (cephalalgia), or headache, has been given significant consideration. The relationship of the sympathetic nervous system to the somatic nervous system has been clarified. The differentiation of the symptomatology thus becomes more clear.

An emphasis on posture, as it relates to cervical and occipital symptomatic pathology, has been considered worthy of a complete chapter.

Newer concepts of pain production relating both peripherally and centrally, to nociceptor theory have been updated. This becomes more meaningful when considering chronic pain of cervical etiology.

Cervical *tension* in this discussion becomes an understandable and treatable clinical entity. Autonomic nervous system control via the spindle system is introduced as a consideration in cervical conditions.

The whiplash condition is fully documented as to etiology, mechanism, nociceptors irritation, and meaningful treatment. The basis for this diagnosis is justified and explained for the physician, the therapist, the judicial system, and the insurance carrier.

Trauma to the cervical spine is differentiated as to (1) hyperextension-hyperflexion injury, (2) posture, and (3) tension. The pathophysiology is fully discussed, enabling therapeutic approaches to be physiologic and effective.

All treatment modalities are discussed and illustrated. A complete, significant, and effective treatment program is outlined, justified, and illustrated for use by the diagnostician, therapist, and the patient. Numerous new illustrations are supplied in this edition, in addition to a new how-to approach.

The disk is fully discussed and its place in cervical symptomatology is explained. Discussion and amplification of this topic clarifies much of what has been thought of as puzzling.

Arthritis is discussed, giving meaning to the role of degeneration and its pathologic causation of pain and impairment.

Extraspinal soft tissue entities such as myofascial pain, scalene entities, and so forth, are fully discussed as well.

This new edition is updated with an extensive bibliography. It is also amply supplied with many new illustrations of the style and quality of previous editions.

RENE CAILLIET, M.D.

Preface to
Second Edition

Over the years since the first edition of *Neck and Arm Pain* there have been numerous additions and changes in diagnostic procedures and in treatment concepts of these syndromes. The second edition is presented in an attempt to update these newer concepts.

Cervical myelopathy was omitted from the previous edition and neglected a very important consideration of painful, disabling aspects of cervical spine disease. The frequency of cervical spondylosis causing myelopathy yet being unrecognized encouraged me to add this important chapter to the second edition.

Numerous concepts of treatment, both surgical and nonsurgical, always benefit from careful review and revision. Numerous theories of local pain and referred pain are always being reviewed clinically and in research laboratories and their pertinence to clinical application needs to be reviewed for the busy clinician who has too little time to assimilate and make applicable these many factions of a common clinical syndrome.

The medical-legal aspect of painful and disabling conditions is continually mandating better medical evaluation and patient care. A better educated patient population also expects better informed medical care delivery as well as explanation of a painful, disabling condition.

The following statement by a legal specialist in a medical journal well summarizes these thoughts:

> Cervical trauma is one of those areas of physical injury which, like head and back injuries, often results in subjective complaints that are extremely difficult for the courts, industrial commissioners, insurance carriers and attorneys to properly evaluate. Leading neurosurgical and orthopedic specialists tell us that there is still much that is unknown about the pathology of cervical trauma, that many times they do not know exactly what to look for in injuries to this area, and that they usually cannot deny subjective complaints in view of lack of precise information.[*]

[*]Allen, WS: Medical-legal aspects of cervical trauma. Clin Neurosurg 2:106–13, 1954.

This revision has been prepared in an attempt to add to this knowledge. It is always with the idea that specialists will also benefit but, more importantly, that students, interns, residents of all specialties, and practitioners of every field of medicine will acquire a sufficient knowledgeable basis for evaluation and treatment of the patient suffering from cervical spine pathology. This is the purpose of the second edition of *Neck and Arm Pain*.

RENE CAILLIET, M.D.

Contents

Illustrations

Introduction

Painful disabling conditions of the cervical spine, and even surgical intervention for cervical spine disease, are rooted in antiquity. Painful disabling conditions of the cervical spine were noted and described in the Middle Ages. The *Papyrus,* written 4600 years ago, is considered to be one of the original orthopedic papers. It contains descriptions of many osseous conditions of the cervical spine. The *Papyrus* was sold to Edwin Smith in 1862 and was translated by Breasted in 1930.

Among the topics listed in the *Papyrus* were vertebral dislocations and sprains. This dissertation actually differentiated cord injuries into upper cervical and lower cervical levels, with appropriate nerve root involvement from specific cervical level.

In antiquity, Tutankhamen described possibly the first cervical laminectomy. In 460 B.C., Hippocrates postulated the occurrence of paralysis from vertebral injuries. He was one of the originators of therapeutic cervical traction and the statement "No head injury, however trivial, should be regarded lightly" is attributed to him. His admonition also applied to injuries of the cervical spine.

Bontecou in 1187 reduced fractures by the application of traction, supplied by adhesive tape, to the patient's face. Crutchfield introduced tongs for traction in 1923.

In the second century A.D., Galen, then the physician to Emperor Marcus Aurelius, incised the cervical cord at interlaminar spaces and noted the specific resultant motor and sensory losses and root levels. Paul of Aegina (625–690 A.D.), a Greek physician, performed cervical laminectomies for spinal cord injuries caused by bony protrusions into the canal.

Later, Ambrose Pare (1559) reduced spinal dislocations with traction and surgically removed osteophytes causing spinal cord compression. Fabricus Hildanus (1646) reduced spinal fracture/dislocation with traction applied to the cervical spine via forceps applied to the neck.

The medical literature contains an increasing number of articles regarding the cervical spine since these dates. The neck-head injury termed *whiplash* was named by Crowe in 1928. This condition was attributed to soft tissue (ligamentous) injuries as a sequela of neck hyperextension beyond the physiologic limits of the neck-head motion.

These conditions are still pertinent in today's society, and some have been aggravated by the addition of motor vehicles and occupational mechanical appliances. Medical science has made advances in diagnosis and treatment. Much remains to be learned but it is the initial evaluation of the condition that leads to the proper diagnosis and appropriate tests. Relevant treatment based on complete knowledge of the impaired functional anatomy leading to pain and impairment should follow. The tissue site of pain production must be recognized.

The newer diagnostic procedures must supplement the diagnostic approach but must never replace the proper interpretation of a careful history, the reproduction of the symptoms during the examination, or the performance of a meaningful orthopedic and neurologic examination.

This text is offered to summarize all of these considerations with the intent of ascertaining proper management of the patient with pain in the neck or from the neck. Acute pain must be remedied, recurrent pain must be prevented, and chronic pain must be avoided.

CHAPTER 1

Functional Anatomy

TOTAL SPINAL COLUMN

The entire spinal column has four superincumbent curves. The curves are termed lordosis or kyphosis, depending upon whether the convexity is anterior or posterior. Lordosis is found in the cervical and lumbar segments, where the convexity of the curve is anterior. Kyphosis is found in the thoracic spine and in the fused vertebrae of the sacrum, where the convexity of the curve is posterior.

All four curves are subservient to the center of gravity (Fig. 1–1). A plumb line, the center of gravity, passes from the external meatus of the ear, transects the odontoid process of the axis (C-2), then transects the bodies of T-1 and T-12. The center of gravity then passes through the sacral promontory, courses slightly posterior to the center of the hip joint, descends anterior to the center of the knee joint, then through the calcaneocuboid joint of the foot, and passes slightly anterior to the lateral malleolei.

A similar relationship of the vertebral column exists when the column is viewed from the front to the back. The center of gravity plumb line descends from the center of the foramen magnum of the skull passes along the posterior superior spinous processes of each vertebra, and passes the tip of the sacrococcyx to a point midway between the two navicular bones of the feet (Fig. 1–2).

CERVICAL SPINE

Viewed laterally from C-1 to C-7, the cervical spine forms a partially symmetrical curve, a lordosis. There may be a sharper curve at the C-5 to C-7 level. Above the atlas, C-1, the head at the occipitocervical level forms a sharp angle to permit the head to be on a horizontal plane.

When viewed anteroposteriorly, the cervical spine may tilt the head slightly

1

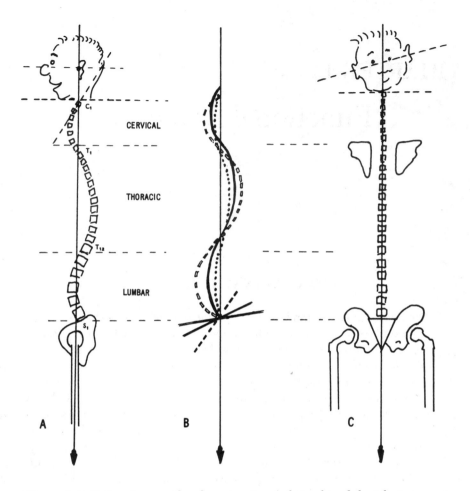

Figure 1–1. Static spine considered erect posture (relationship of physiologic curves to plumb line of gravity). (*A*) Lateral view of erect posture, (*B*) change of superincumbent curves influenced by change of sacral angle, (*C*) anteroposterior plumb-line view with head tilted slightly to one side.

to one side. This may be explained by the facets of the occiput, atlas, and axis being slightly asymmetrical.

Viewed laterally, the composite alignment of all four spinal curves, depicts the erect posture of the individual. The subject of posture will be discussed fully later in chapter 3.

The cervical spine supports the head, allowing precise movement and position. All vital nerve centers are in the head allowing controlled vision, vestibular balance, auditory direction, and olfactory nerves; essentially it controls all conscious neuromuscular functions. The head atop the cervical spine must be

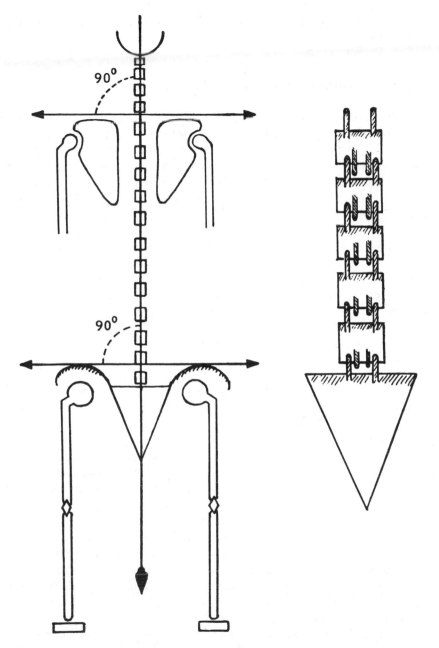

Figure 1–2. Spinal alignment from anteroposterior aspect, anteroposterior view of the erect human spine. With both legs equal in length, the spine supports the pelvis in a level horizontal plane, and the spine, taking off at a right angle (90-degree), ascends in a straight line. The facets shown in the enlarged drawing on the right show their parallel alignment and proper symmetry in this erect position.

supported in the appropriate position to allow for specific motion to accomplish its functions.

Cervical Spine Functional Units

The cervical spine is an aggregate of superimposed *functional units,* each comprises of two adjacent vertebral bodies. Below the second vertebra, C-2, the axis, each unit has adjacent vertebrae separated by intervertebral disks. The third, fourth, fifth, and sixth vertebrae are similar and conform to what can be termed *typical* functional units. The remaining vertebral units are unique.

To functionally evaluate the cervical spine, it can be divided into an upper cervical segment (above C-3) and a lower cervical segment (C-3 to C-7). Each of these segments functions differently.

The functional unit of the cervical spine can be divided into two columns: the anterior column, composed of the vertebrae, their longitudinal ligaments, and the interposed disks; and the posterior columns containing the neural osseous canal, the posterior ligaments, the zygapophyseal joints, and the erector muscles of the spine (Holdsworth, White and Panjabi).

Anatomically, the intervertebral foramina are located between these two sagittal columns. Conceptionally, the anterior (flexor) cervical muscles are not included in this designation but rightfully belong to the anterior column.

Another depiction of the cervical spine has been postulated in which the spine is divided into three columns (Louis). The anterior column is composed of the vertebrae and the disks, whereas one posterior column is divided into the lamina, the pedicles, and the spinous processes and the other column is composed of the zygapophyseal (facet) joints.

The purpose of this division is to clarify the physiologic movement and to discern the pathologic deviations that result in pain and dysfunction.

The cervical spine moves physiologically in specific directions as dictated by the planes of the articulations moving from center-of-gravity coordinates (White and Panjabi). Movement can be listed as flexion, extension, lateral flexion, and rotation. Forces of vertical compression must also be equated. Each segment of the cervical spine thus has possible physiologic movements and has movement restricted by the design of the intrinsic structure of that specific segment, especially of the articular planes. There are also restrictions imposed upon articular motion, in direction and extent, by the annular fibers, ligaments, muscles, and joint capsules.

Cervical Vertebrae: Lower Cervical Segment. A typical cervical vertebrae (C-3 to C-7) has specific characteristics. The anterior width is greater than the posterior width. The width of the intervertebral disk is similar, wider anteriorly than posteriorly (Fig. 1–3). The difference in width accounts partly for the cervical lordotic curve (Fig. 1–4).

The cervical vertebral body is 50 percent wider transversely than it is an-

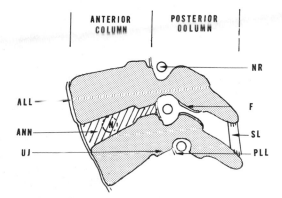

Figure 1–3. Lateral view of a functional unit of the cervical spine C 3 to C-7. The spine is divided into anterior and posterior columns. The component parts are ALL=anterior longitudinal ligament, ANN=annulus fibrosus, UJ=uncovertebral joint, NR=nerve root, F=facet, SL= superior ligament, PLL= posterior longitudinal ligament.

teroposteriorly. The superior surface is concave from side to side due in part to the presence of uncinate processes (the uncovertebral bodies). These processes are also termed *Luschka's joints*. The inferior surface of the vertebral body is concave anterioposteriorly and convex laterally (Fig. 1–5). The transverse processes are located on both sides of the vertebral bodies. They are regarded as developmental ribs. Located within each transverse process is a foramen through which traverse the vertebral arteries (see Fig. 1–5). The transverse bodies contain gutters along which the spinal nerves traverse; these gutters run laterally and anteriorly.

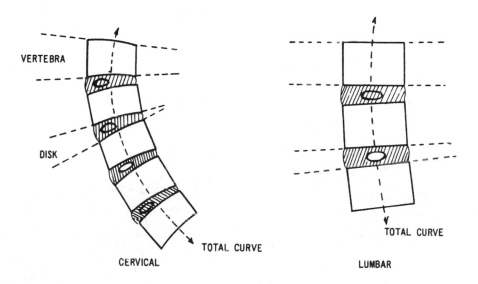

Figure 1–4. Comparative curves of cervical and lumbar spine related to disk shapes.

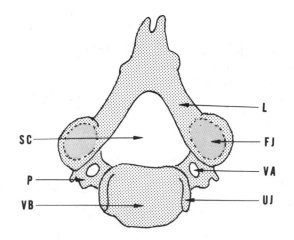

Figure 1–5. When viewed from above (superior view) the typical cervical vertebra (C-3 to C-7) is composed of the following elements: L=lamina, FJ=facet joint, VA=vertebral artery (foramen), UJ=uncovertebral joint (Luschka), SC=spinal canal, P=pedicle, VB=vertebral body.

Between two adjacent vertebrae, caudally from C-2, there are found intervertebral disks. These disks, as has been noted, are wider anteriorly than posteriorly. Each disk is composed of an annulus and a nucleus (Fig. 1–6). Each disk has a soft inner structure, the nucleus pulposus, now simply called the nucleus. The nucleus is surrounded by 12 lamellae, each approximately 1 mm thick. The

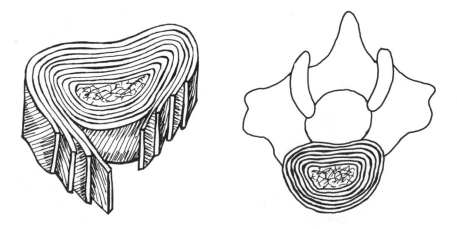

Figure 1–6. Annulus fibrosus. (*Left*) Layer concept of annulus fibrosus. (*Right*) Circumferential annular fibers around the central, pulpy nucleus (nucleus pulposus).

laminae are formed by sheets of collagen fibers that attach from adjacent vertebrae endplates and course diagonally to the opposite vertebral endplates. The annular fibers run at angulations in the periphery of the disk different from those in the centrum near the nucleus (Fig. 1–7). The boundary between the inner annular layer and the nucleus is not clearly defined and forms a transition zone (Hukins). The superior and inferior borders of the disk are the cartilaginous endplates of adjacent vertebrae. Each disk is approximately 1 cm thick, and each endplate is 1 mm thick. Each annular lamella is firmly attached to the vertebral bodies and their endplates.

The intervertebral disks have a vascular supply from birth until approximately the second decade of life, when the blood vessels become obliterated by calcification of the vertebral endplates. By the third decade the disk is avascular.

With onset of avascularity, the nutrition of the disk is by diffusion of dialysates through the endplates and imbibition from osmotic gradients of the dissolved ions within the disk substance.

There is also a mechanical factor to imbibition. As the disk becomes compressed, it expresses fluid, and as it is released, it imbibes. This alternate compression-relaxation allows the disk to imbibe in a spongelike manner. The elasticity of the annular fibers and the compressibility of the nucleus allow this mechanical imbibitory action.

The nucleus is a highly hydrated (80 percent water) proteoglycan gel containing some finely dispersed collagen fibers (less than 5 percent). This proteoglycan gel contains many negatively charged sulphate groups that attract and bind water and prevent outward diffusion. The nucleus is completely contained within an annular tube which maintains its intrinsic pressure (Fig. 1–8).

The self-contained hydrated nucleus conforms to the laws of fluid under pressure. The gel cannot be compressed; it can be merely reformed so long as the container is elastic. Any external pressure applied to a liquid at any point is transmitted equally in all directions (in the annulus, in this case) according to Pascal's law (1623–62).

The annulus is composed of sheets of parallel collagen fibers. The oblique direction of the collagen fibers forming the outer layers runs in the opposite direction to the collagen fibers of the next inner layer. Each layer (sheet) has alternating direction of the collagen fibers in the sheets. The collagen fibers are surrounded, essentially contained within, layers of hydrated proteoglycan gel, which lubricate and nutritionally support the collagen fibrils.

The manner in which the annular fibers attach to the endplates and interface with each layer permits movement of the adjacent vertebrae within a functional unit, allowing flexion, extension, and a slight degree of rotation (Fig. 1–9).

Each collagen fiber is a trihelix chain of numerous amino acids. Each amino acid is connected to its adjacent acid component, forming a springlike fiber. This fiber allows elongation but, since it allows only the elongation of the coiled fiber, it has limited extensibility. (Fig. 1–10).

Neck motion, occurring by movement of each cervical functional unit, is

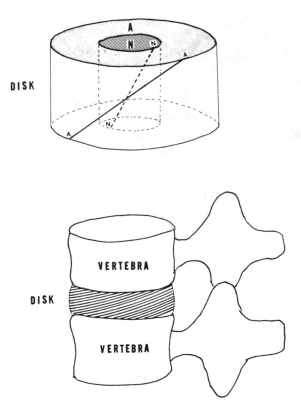

Figure 1–7. Annular fiber, (*top*) a schematic analysis of the intervertebral disk within the functional unit, (*bottom*). A=annulus; and N=nucleus. There are the same number of collagen fibers in the outer sheath (A◄——►A) and in the inner sheath (N◄——►N). The difference is in their angulation and length.

restricted by the limited elasticity of the annular fibers of each intervertebral annulus. The mobility of the functional unit is also limited by the presence of the longitudinal ligaments, which attach from the cranium to each vertebra caudally down to the sacrum. The anterior longitudinal ligaments are firmly attached to each vertebra, and the posterior longitudinal ligaments are more sparsely attached. These long ligaments are essentially the outer layers of each intervertebral disk annulus.

The ligaments are composed of parallel layers of collagen fibers with limited proteoglycan matrix. The collagen fibers of these ligaments are less tortuous and, because of their parallel attachment, have less elongation potential.

Flexion is limited by the posterior longitudinal ligament, the posterior intervertebral ligaments which attach to the transverse processes and the posterior superior spine, and also by the limited elasticity of the fascia of the extensor

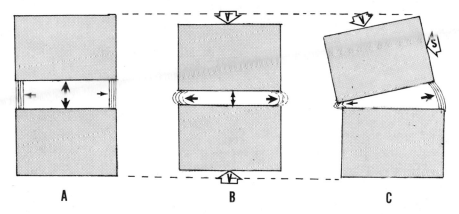

Figure 1–8. Hydraulic mechanism of the intervertebral disk. (*A*) Normal resting disk. Internal pressure is equalized in all directions; annular fibers taut, vertebrae distracted. (*B*) Compressed disk from external forces or muscular tension; nucleus deforms and annular fibers bulge. (*C*) Flexion of functional unit. The disk is compressed on the concave side and separated on the convex side. The annular fibers elongate to allow this. The superior vertebra shears slightly in flexion (arrow *S*).

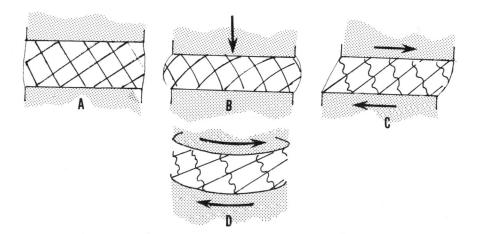

Figure 1–9. Elasticity of annular fibers in vertebral movements. (*A*) With no movement and the vertebrae separated, all the layers of annular fibers are taut. (*B*) With external compression, the disk bulges but the fibers remain taut, albeit curved. (*C*) With transitional shear, the fibers in the direction of shear are stretched, and the opposing fibers become relaxed. (*D*) With rotation, the fibers in the direction of rotation become elongated and the other layer fibers become slack. All annular fibers elongate to their respective elasticity.

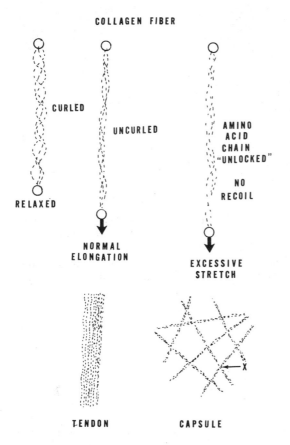

COLLAGEN FIBER

CURLED

UNCURLED

RELAXED

NORMAL
ELONGATION

AMINO
ACID
CHAIN
"UNLOCKED"

NO
RECOIL

EXCESSIVE
STRETCH

TENDON

CAPSULE

X

Figure 1–10. Collagen fiber. Each collagen fiber is a trihelix chain of amino acids chemically (electrically) bound together. The fibers uncurl to their physiologic length, then recoil when the elongation force is released. If the collagen fiber is elongated past its physiologic length, the amino acid chains become disrupted, and the fiber no longer returns to its resting length.

A tendon consists of parallel bands of collagen fibers. In a capsule, the collagen fibers crisscross and glide over each other at their intersection (X). The capsule depicted here elongates as far as each collagen fiber permits.

musculature.

Excessive extension of the functional units is limited by the direct contact of the laminae, the facets, and the posterosuperior spinous process.

The primary function of the cervical spine is to support the head and to allow movement in every direction needed for its neurophysiologic functions. Structurally the cervical spine is well constructed to accomplish all these functions.

All movements of the cervical spine are a composite of primary segmental motion (Fig. 1–11). It is well documented that motion on merely one plane is not possible, but is a combination of movements in several directions. For example, flexion and extension also have some gliding, lateral motion and also include rotation.

Within the upper cervical segment, the occipito-atlas-axis segment, a greater degree of motion is possible. Total neck movement, however, demands participation of *all* the cervical vertebral segments. Each joint employs total motion allowed by the articular configuration, the elasticity of the ligaments, the muscles, and the annular fibers. Passive motion is thereby assured. Physiologic active motion implies that there is also intact, or at least adequate, muscular action, indicating sufficient innervation with good central nervous system control.

Any of these physiologic restrictive tissues may be altered with the loss of a segment as well as total range of motion from structural damage or from the intrusion of pain from motion.

Their significant structural differences encourage dividing the cervical spine into *upper* and *lower* cervical segments. There is also a rational basis for differentiating between the *static* cervical spine and the *kinetic* cervical spine.

The greater number of cervical vertebral functional units are contained in the lower segment, and it is from this segment that nerve roots emerge to supply the upper extremities.

The lower cervical segment begins from the inferior border of the axis (C-2) where this vertebra articulates with the C-3 vertebra. Flexion and extension of C-2 upon C-3 occurs between the articular facets of the body of C-2 and the upper facets of C-3. This motion occurs as a gliding or rocking motion.

Rotation of the second cervical vertebra (C-2) upon the third vertebra (C-3) is mechanically limited by the structures of the adjacent vertebrae as well as by the constraints of the intervertebral disk annular fibers and the ligaments. The anterior tip of the upper articular process of the third cervical vertebra (C-3) impinges upon the lateral process of the second cervical vertebra (C-2) (Fig. 1–12).

From the third cervical vertebra caudally, the cervical spine comprises contiguous functional units of similar structural design.

Motion in this segment includes flexion, extension, lateral flexion, rotation, and composite movement of these primary motions. As has been stated, few motions occur in only one plane; most motions are composites. It has been confirmed that in a long elastic tubular structure there can be no lateral flexion without commensurate rotation. The opposite is also true, that is, there can be no rotation of a flexible tubular structure without some lateral motion (Lovett).

Motion of a functional unit in any direction causes some distortion of the intervertebral disk. This distortion engenders some elongation of the annular fibers when the total disk deforms, whether in flexion, extension, lateral motion, or rotation.

In forward flexion, the anterior disk space undergoes compression with a simultaneous separation of the posterior elements. In forward flexion there also occurs a forward gliding motion of the superior vertebra upon the contiguous inferior vertebra (Fig. 1–13).

The intervertebral disk contained within the anterior column compresses anteriorly and widens posteriorly. This flexion is accompanied by some anterior shear. Along with anterior flexion and shear of the disk there is separation and some shear motion of the posterior column structures.

Excessive elongation of the posterior annular fibers of the disk in flexion is also limited by the posterior longitudinal ligament. The alignment of the collagen fibers within the long ligaments has been discussed. The alignment and the

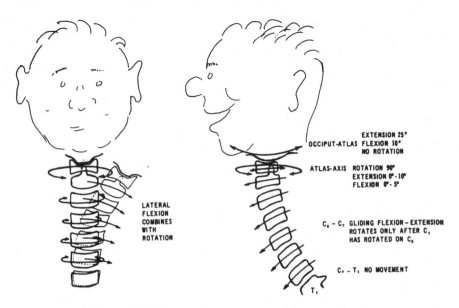

Figure 1–11. Composite movements of the cervical spine.

rangement of the annular sheets of collagen fibers permit this flexion to their physiologic limits and, when these limits are reached, invoke the restriction of the long ligament. This limitation of elongation of annular fibers prevents disruption of the uncoiled annular collagen fibers.

Excessive flexion beyond physiologic limits is also resisted by the interspinous and posterior spinous ligaments as well as by the elasticity of the erector

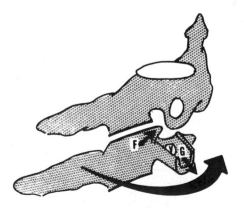

Figure 1–12. Rotation of C-2 upon C-3 is limited by the mechanical locking of the articular structures. The anterior tip of the upper articular process of C-3 impinges upon the lateral margin of the foramen of the vertebral artery (V). The nerve root of C_3 emerges through the gutter (G).

Figure 1–13. Flexion of a typical functional unit in the lower cervical segment (C-3 to C-7) finds the superior gliding forward upon the inferior vertebra. The anterior disk space (A) narrows and the posterior elements (P) separate. The intervertebral foramen (F) opens in the flexion motion of the cervical spine.

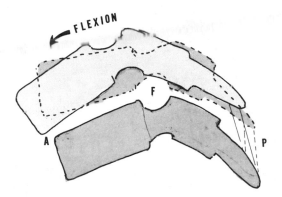

spinae muscle fascia.

In cervical spine extension (sometimes called posterior flexion), the posterior aspect of the disk compresses, and the anterior portion elongates. This motion is again limited by the anterior longitudinal ligaments as well as by the elasticity of the annular fibers.

In extension, the posterior zygapophyseal (facet) joints glide posteriorly in a sagittal downward direction. The degree of extension is limited (Fig. 1–14) by gradual approximation of the facet surfaces as well as by the elasticity of the articular capsules.

Foraminal Opening. In cervical flexion, the laminae separate and the intervertebral foramina *open*. The pedicles separate as the superior facets glide forward and upward (Fig. 1–15). Similarly, upon extension of the neck, the foramina *close* (narrow). In lateral flexion (obviously with some rotation to that

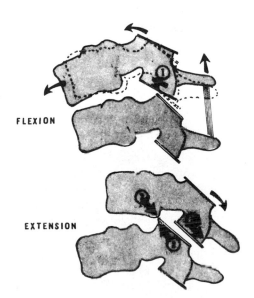

Figure 1–14. Translatory gliding on cervical flexion. The superior facet glides forward (1) and the essentially vertical facet elevates the posterior element until the interspinous ligament stops the movement. In extension, the superior facet glides posteriorly (3) until the inferior facet impinges upon the vertebra (2) and stops extension.

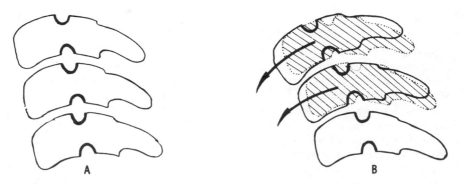

Figure 1–15. Gliding movement in flexing spine from C-3 through C-7. (*A*) Neutral position. (*B*) Flexion with forward gliding, anterior disk compression, and widening posterior space.

side), the foramina close on the side toward which the neck flexes and open on the side away from which the neck flexes (Fig. 1–16).

The cervical spinal canal has a specific length in the neutral position which is determined by the genetic structure, the width of the vertebrae, the width of the intervertebral disks, and the physiologic curvature in each individual. As the neck flexes forward, the canal lengthens. Similarly, as the neck extends (posterior flexion), the length of the canal shortens (Fig. 1–17).

The spinal cord contained within the canal must, therefore, also elongate upon flexion and shorten upon cervical extension. This alteration in the length of the cord is possible by virtue of the *plasticity* of the spinal cord. The dural sheath of the spinal cord and of the nerve root sleeves does not have this plasticity but has *elasticity* by virtue of its being plicated (Fig. 1–18).

The relationship of the nerve roots and their dural sheath within the intervertebral foramina will be discussed in detail in chapter 2, The Cervical Nerves.

Cervical Vertebrae: Upper Cervical Segment. There are essentially five articulations in the upper cervical segment: occipital-atlas-axis joints. There are two joints formed by the opposing lateral masses of the atlas with the occiput and two joints between the lateral masses of the axis. The fifth joint is between the posterior surface of the arch of the atlas and the anterior surface of the odontoid process and the transverse ligament of the atlas.

Occipital-Axis Joint. The occiput articulates upon the atlas with the inferior convex condyles of the cranium moving upon the two superior concave facets of the lateral bodies of the atlas (C-1).

The movement in this articulation is that of flexion-extension in the sagittal plane. This is essentially the movement used when nodding *yes* (Fig. 1–19). Flexion occurs through a range of 10 degrees with an extension of 25 degrees, a total of 35 degrees. Due to the configuration of the condyles, *no* significant lateral flexion or rotation occurs.

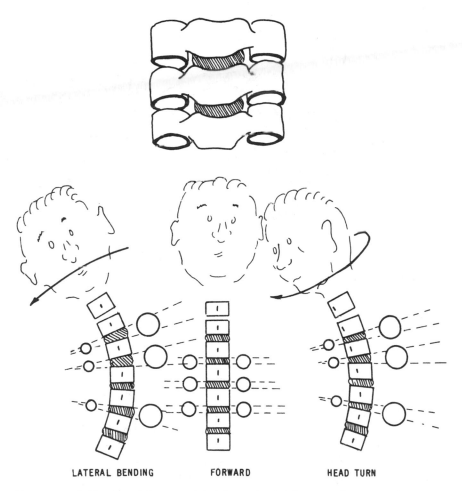

LATERAL BENDING   FORWARD   HEAD TURN

Figure 1–16. Foraminal closure in head during lateral flexion and turning. The foramina close on the side toward which the head rotates or bends laterally, and they open on the opposite side.

Atlas: First Cervical Vertebra (C-1). The first cervical vertebra, termed the *atlas,* possesses no typical vertebral body. In place of a central body it contains two lateral masses connected by anterior and posterior arches (Fig. 1–20). As stated, the superior surface of the atlas lateral body is concave and articulates with the condyles of the occiput.

The interior surfaces of the lateral atlas bodies articulate with the superior facets of the lateral bodies of the axis. The surfaces of the lateral masses of the atlas-axis joints incline laterally and downward, allowing flexion extension in the sagittal plane and restriction of lateral or rotatory motion.

The inferior surfaces of the atlas are concave in relation to the convexity of

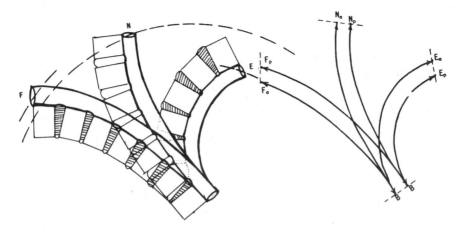

Figure 1–17. Alteration in spinal canal length. Length of neutral (N) spinal canal compared with that in flexion (F) and extension (E). In flexion the canal is longer and the anterior wall (F_a–B) is shorter than the posterior wall (F_p–B). In extension the total length of the canal is shorter, with the anterior (E_a–B) longer than the posterior wall (E_p–B). In neutral position both walls of the canal (N_a–B and N_p–B) are equal.

the superior surfaces of the axis. This allows rotation in the sagittal plane as well as axial rotation about the axis of the odontoid.

There are no intervertebral disks between these upper cervical functional units. These joints are synarthrosis in that they are collagen-fibrous capsules.

On the posterior surface of the anterior arch of the atlas is a small facet that articulates with the odontoid process (dens).

Axis: Second Cervical Vertebra (C-2). The axis (Fig. 1–21) also has no central vertebral body as in a typical vertebra. This vertebra has two lateral masses that contain superior and inferior facetal surfaces. These lateral masses are connected by anterior and posterior arches. The anterior arch is thickened centrally, forming a body from which projects superiorly the odontoid process. The central body descends to form an articulation with the central body of the C-3 vertebra.

The lateral masses articulate with the lateral bodies of the atlas superiorly. The inferior surfaces articulate with the C-3 vertebra. There are interspinal ligaments that connect and limit the motion between these vertebrae.

A major ligament is the transverse ligament of the atlas, which seats the odontoid process, allowing rotation between these two vertebrae (Fig. 1–22). Rotation of 45 degrees to the left and rotation of 45 degrees to the right is possible: a total rotation of approximately 90 degrees. Some flexion and extension are possible but are very slight.

Rotation of the next lower functional units C-2 upon C-3 is mechanically limited by a bony locking mechanism in which the anterior tip of the superior articular process of C-3 impinges upon the lateral process of the axis (Fig. 1–23).

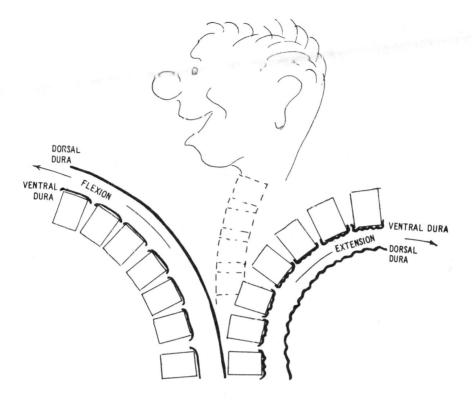

Figure 1–18. Reaction of the dura in neck flexion and extension. The dura becomes taut in physiologic tension during flexion, thus "ironed out." In extension, the dura folds, or pleats, and apparently shortens (see text). The assumption that the cord *ascends* in the canal during flexion and *descends* during extension (carrying the nerve roots with it) is proven.

There are foramina in the transverse bodies of the upper cervical vertebrae through which pass the vertebral arteries. At the C-2 level, the artery makes a sharp angulation. The artery is protected from excessive rotation by the locking mechanism described above.

Ligaments of the Upper Cervical Segment. The ligaments of the atlantoaxial joints deserve particular attention inasmuch as they allow specific motion, albeit limited: the limit to motion protects the contents or the spinal canal (spinal cord and nerve roots) against damage in the case of severe external trauma.

The transverse ligament arises from two small tubercles on both sides of the anterior arch of the atlas and from the posterior aspects of the lateral masses of the atlas (Fig. 1–24). This ligament crosses the spinal canal and forms a sling holding the odontoid process against the anterior arch. Ascending superiorly

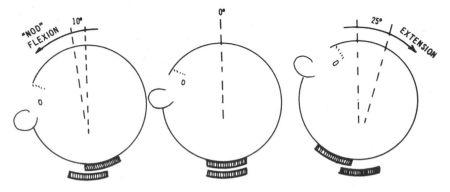

Figure 1–19. Occipital-atlas movement. Flexion-extension gliding of occiput on atlas in a nodding motion. No rotation or lateral flexion is possible.

from the midpoint of the transverse ligament is a ligament that attaches to the margin of the foramen magnum. There is also a descending ligament from this midpoint that attaches to the axis. These branching ligaments form a cross. (Fig. 1–25).

Under the transverse ligament a small ligament arises from the tip of the odontoid and attaches to the margin of the foramen magnum. This ligament is known as the apical (suspensory) ligament (see Fig. 1–24).

Descending from the condyles of the occipital bone are two ligaments that merge upon the odontoid process; known as alar ligaments (see Fig. 1–24). Their primary function is to limit rotation of the occiput and the atlas upon the axis. They also prevent lateral subluxation of the occiput-atlas on the axis.

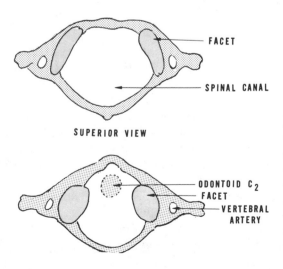

Figure 1–20. The atlas (C-1) is viewed from above and below. The upper facets articulate with the condyles of the occiput and the inferior facets articulate with the superior facets of the axis (C-2). The odontoid (dens) of C-2 articulates with a small facet in the central area of the anterior arch.

Figure 1–21. The axis (C-2) is the second vertebra. The superior facets articulate as a synarthrosis with the inferior facets of the atlas (C-1). The inferior facets articulate with the superior facets of the third vertebra (C-3). The odontoid process (the dens) ascends within the spinal canal of the atlas. It is held firmly by the transverse ligaments.

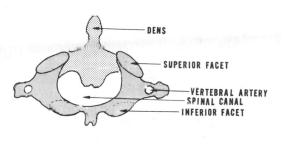

DENS
SUPERIOR FACET
VERTEBRAL ARTERY
SPINAL CANAL
INFERIOR FACET

There are two major ligaments that extend from the inner aspects of the lateral masses of the atlas and descend to attach posterolaterally to the body of the axis. These are termed accessory atlantoaxial ligaments (Fig. 1–26). Their primary purpose is to limit rotation of the atlas upon the axis.

The posterior longitudinal ligament, which descends from the foramen magnum caudally to ultimately attach to the sacrum in the cervical spine attaches and descends from the posterior surfaces of the vertebral bodies anterior to the spinal cord. The posterior longitudinal ligament fans out at its attachment to the occipital bone. This portion of the ligament is termed the *tectorial ligament*.

There are other smaller yet powerful ligaments that interconnect these three cervical vertebrae, just as there are strong capsular structures that contain the lateral body articulations.

The *posterior longitudinal ligaments* that extend from each posterior spinous process essentially restrict excessive flexion (Fig. 1–27).

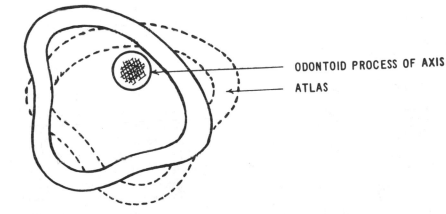

ODONTOID PROCESS OF AXIS

ATLAS

Figure 1–22. Rotation of the atlas about the odontoid process of the axis (C-1 around C-2).

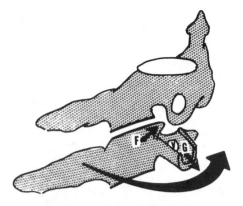

Figure 1–23. Rotation of C-2 upon C-3 is limited by the mechanical locking of the articular structures. The anterior tip of the upper articular process of C-3 impinges upon the lateral margin of the foramen of the vertebral artery (*V*). The nerve root of C-3 emerges through the gutter (*G*).

The *ligamentum flavum* extends from the posterior arch of the atlas to the surface of the lamina of the axis. It assists in preventing forward subluxation of the occiput-atlas upon the axis.

The *ligamentum nuchae* is an interspinous ligament that extends from the occiput, attaching to each posterior spinous process as it descends (Fig. 1–28). It reinforces the posterior aspect of the neck and acts as a septum dividing the extensor muscles of the neck.

Ligamentous Function. The cervical ligaments have been enumerated and dilineated, but it would be of value here to ascertain their specific functions.

The transverse ligament holds the odontoid process into the notch located posteriorly in the center of the anterior arch. This allows the head and atlas to rotate to the right and to the left. It also maintains the odontoid process in the anterior portion of the spinal canal and ensures adequate room for the spinal cord.

Should there be any injury or disease that disrupts or elongates the transverse ligament, the odontoid process can move posteriorly and encroach upon

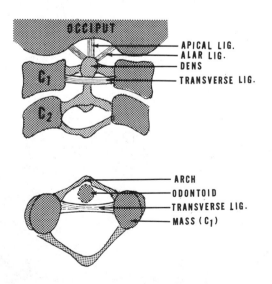

Figure 1–24. Occipital-atlas-axis ligaments: The ligaments that support this portion of the upper cervical segment are the apical ligaments (from the tip of the dens to the foramen magnum) and the alar ligament (also from the dens cephalad). The transverse ligament acts as a sling holding the dens against the posterior aspect of the anterior arch of the atlas.

Figure 1–25. Transverse or cross ligaments: Attached from the medial aspects of the bodies of the atlas, the transverse ligament crosses the spinal canal and forms the support of the odontoid dens process. Arising from the superior aspect of this ligament ascends a ligament that attaches to the foramen magnum. A similar ligament descends to attach to the axis.

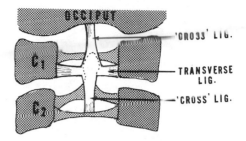

the spinal cord. This can be seen in standard x-ray examinations that depict the lateral view of the cervical spine with the head flexed (bending forward). The degree of cord encroachment is determined clinically by performing a neurologic examination and discovering the presence of upper motor neuron signs. A magnetic resonance image (MRI) also can be diagnostic.

The alar ligaments limit rotation and also restrict lateral motion of the odontoid process. If one of the alar ligaments is severed, the head and atlas can sublux laterally.

The accessory atlantoaxial ligaments limit the degree of rotation of the head upon the atlas and the atlas upon the axis. The impairment of one accessory ligament will allow excessive rotation to the opposite side. This can be determined by x-ray studies through the open mouth, taken with rotation of the head in both directions.

The alar and accessory ligaments are short ligaments attached to two adjacent bony structures and are thus susceptible to injury. Excessive, forceful, or abrupt rotation may be the causative factor in sustained ligamentous injury.

Musculature of the Neck. The neck muscles can be divided functionally into two major groups: those that flex and extend the head upon the spine and those that flex and extend the entire remaining cervical spine. The former are termed the *capital movers*, the latter the *cervical movers* (Fig. 1–29).

The capital flexors are principally the short recti and longus capitis. The capital extensors are four short muscles that extend from the base of the skull to attach to the atlas (C-1) and axis (C-2). These muscles include the posterior rectus capitis minor and major and the obliquus capitis superior and inferior.

The longer muscles, splenius capitis and splenius cervicis are primarily ro-

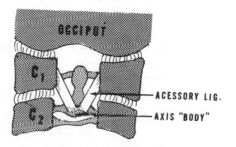

Figure 1–26. Accessory atlanto–axial ligaments. Two ligaments attach from the medial aspects of the bodies of the atlas and descend to converge upon the body of the axis anterior to the odontoid process.

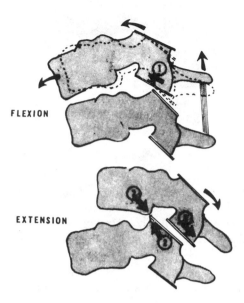

FLEXION

EXTENSION

Figure 1–27. Translatory gliding on cervical flexion. The superior facet glides forward (1) and the essentially vertical facet elevates the posterior element until the interspinous ligament stops the movement. In extension, the superior facet glides posteriorly (3) until the inferior facet impinges upon the vertebra (2) and stops further extension.

tators of the head but are also extensors when they contract bilaterally. There are other longer muscles of the upper thoracic spine and scapulae that extend the cervical spine, rotate it, and flex it laterally. These include the trapezius, levator scapulae, and others.

The main mass of neck muscles is located in the extensor portion of the upper cervical segment: the atlantoaxial area (Fig. 1–30). This indicates the need for strong muscles in that cervical region to guard against trauma. The greatest bulk of flexor muscles is located at the midcervical region (C-4 to C-5), which is the region of the lower cervical segment that has the greatest degree of motion and is thus the area of greatest mechanical wear and tear and exposure to trauma and stress.

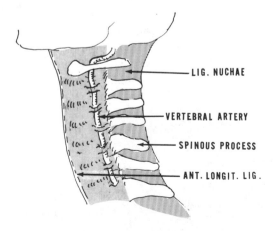

LIG. NUCHAE

VERTEBRAL ARTERY

SPINOUS PROCESS

ANT. LONGIT. LIG.

Figure 1–28. Ligamentum nuchae. This firm ligament attaches from the base of the skull to each posterior superior spinous process throughout the length of the cervical spine. It acts as a septum dividing the erector spinae muscle masses.

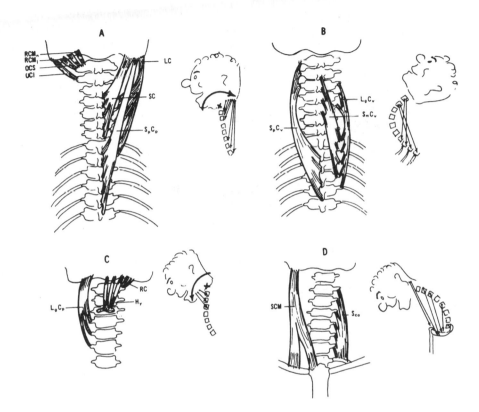

Figure 1–29. Musculature of the head and neck. (A) and (B) The musculature of the extensor mechanism of the head and neck. (A) The capital extensors attach to the skull and move the head upon the neck. (B) The cervical extensors originate and attach upon the cervical spine and alter the curvature of the cervical spine. (C) and (D) Flexion musculature. (C) The capital flexors flex the head upon the neck. (D) The cervical flexors attach exclusively upon cervical vertebrae and have no significant functional attachment to the skull.

RCM_n	=	rectus capitis minor	LC	=	longissimus capitis
RCM_j	=	rectus capitis major	SC	=	semispinalis capitis
OCS	=	obliquus capitis superior	S_pC_p	=	splenius capitis
OCI	=	obliquus capitis inferior	S_pC_v	=	splenius cervicis
L_gC_p	=	longus capitis	L_mC_v	=	longissimus cervicis
RC	=	rectus capitis anterior and laternal	S_mC_v	=	semispinalis cervicis
H_y	=	hyoideus and suprahyoid muscles	SCM	=	sternocleidomastoid
			S_{ca}	=	scalene medius and antieus

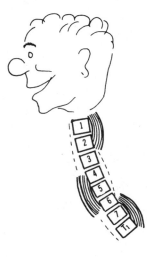

Figure 1–30. Sites of major muscle bulk in the cervical spine. The major bulk of extensor musculature in the head and neck is at the occipital-atlas-axis region and at the last cervical (C-6) thoracic articulations. These sites are the major points of stress. The major anterior (flexor) bulk is at the C4-5 space, implying that the major flexion occurs here. This is also the site of maximum lordosis (curvature).

BIBLIOGRAPHY

Holdsworth, F: Fractures dislocations, and fracture-dislocations of the spine. Current Concepts Rehab Med. 4: fall-winter, 1988.

Hukins, DWL: Disc structure and function. In Ghosh, P (ed): The Biology of the Intervertebral Disc, vol. 1. CRC Press, Boca Raton, Florida, 1988.

Louis, R: Surgery of the Spine. Springer-Verlag, Berlin, 1983.

Lovett, RW: Lateral curvature of the spine and round shoulders. P. Blakiston Son & Co., Philadelphia, 1907.

White, AA and Panjabi, MM: Clinical Biomechanics of the Spine. JB Lippincott, Philadelphia, 1978.

CHAPTER 2

The Cervical Nerves

The nerves of the cervical region, with the formation of the cervicobrachial plexus and the nerves to the head, play such a vital role in the function of the upper extremities and are so involved in the production of pain and impairment that they are discussed separately here.

Each cervical nerve is a spinal nerve formed of the union of the anterior (ventral) motor and posterior (dorsal) sensory nerve fibers that have emerged bilaterally from the spinal cord gray matter (Fig. 2–1). The two emerging fibers of the anterior and posterior roots merge into one larger branch (Fig. 2–2) before leaving the vertebral spinal area to proceed as a peripheral nerve. The emergence differs in the upper cervical area from that in the lower cervical spinal segment.

GREATER SUPERIOR OCCIPITAL NERVE

The upper cervical nerve roots (C_1 to C_2 and a branch of C_3) innervate the head and face and merit separate evaluation. The nerve root C_2 is called the *greater occipital nerve* and is the major source of head and facial pain when it becomes *entrapped,* compressed, stretched, or in any way encroached upon.

Hunter and Mayfield postulated that the C_2 nerve becomes entrapped between the posterior arch of the axis (C-1 vertebra) and the lamina of the axis (C-2) and thus can be damaged when excessive extension of the head with simultaneous rotation to that side occurs. This concept exists in much of the literature on this subject, but is not anatomically feasible (Bogduk).

It has also been claimed that the nerve root C_2—the major branch of the greater occipital nerve—becomes entrapped in its passage through the posterior atlantoaxial membrane. It is also postulated that when this nerve becomes a peripheral nerve, it passes between a small area formed by the site of attach-

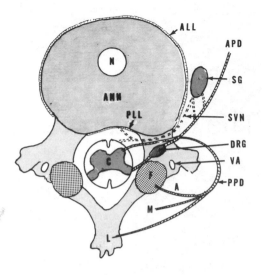

Figure 2–1. Component fibers of a cervical nerve. A view of a functional unit depicts the components of a cervical nerve.

C=spinal cord
SG=stellate ganglion
DRG=dorsal root ganglion
APD=anterior primary division
PPD=posterior primary division
A=articular branch of PPD
M=muscular branch of PPD
L=ligamentous branch of PPD

SVN=sinu vertebral nerve; branches to dura and PLL
N=disk nucleus
ANN=disk annulus
ALL=anterior longitudinal ligament
PLL=posterior longitudinal ligament
F=facet
VA=vertebral artery foramen

ment to the occipital condyles of the upper trapezius muscle and the sterno-cleidomastoid muscles.

The anatomy of this cervical region is now more clearly defined and the nerve and its emergence are portrayed in a more rational manner, helping to clarify much of the controversy in the discussion of head pain of cervical origin (Bogduk).

The C_2 nerve root emerges from the cord fila to pass laterally to the posterior atlantoaxial membrane. The C_2 dorsal root lies deep within the obliquus inferior muscles and is dorsal to the atlantoaxial joint (Fig. 2–3). It is held in that position by fascia attaching it to the capsule of the joint.

The nerve roots then proceed laterally and divide into dorsal and ventral roots at the atlantoaxial joint. The ventral root passes across the atlantoaxial joint capsule being held there by fascia. It proceeds laterally to cross over the vertebral artery (Fig. 2–4).

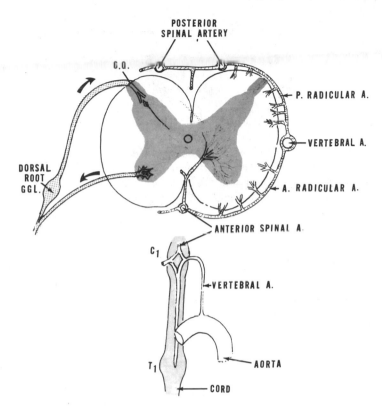

POSTERIOR
SPINAL ARTERY

C.O.

P. RADICULAR A.

VERTEBRAL A.

DORSAL
ROOT
GGL.

A. RADICULAR A.

ANTERIOR SPINAL A.

C_1

VERTEBRAL A.

AORTA

T_1

CORD

Figure 2–2. Formation of nerve root: cross-section of spinal cord. The cross-section of the spinal cord depicts the central gray matter. On the left are the sensory dorsal root ganglia (GGL) and the descending motor root (curved arrows). SG indicates the substantia gelatinosum of the dorsal horn wherein enters the sensory fibers.

On the right are shown the arterial supply of the cord. The vertebral arteries begin at the subclavian arch of the aorta. The vertebral arteries ascend from the arch to branch circumferentially around the cord as anterior and posterior, radicular arteries forming anteriorly the anterior spinal artery and posteriorly the posterior spinal artery.

The lower drawing reveals the arterial cord configuration, with C-1 the atlas and T-1 the first thoracic level.

The dorsal ramus also passes laterally deep to the obliquus inferior muscle ultimately to supply the longissmus capitis, splenius capitis, and semispinal muscles. There are also branches of C_3 dorsal root that merge with this C_2 root.

The greater occipital nerve (C-2 to C-3) curves around the obliquus inferior muscles and penetrates the semispinalis muscle to pierce the scalp soft tissues and ultimately to innervate the scalp (see Fig. 1–21). It penetrates neither the upper trapezius nor the sternocleidomastoid muscle but, rather, emerges in

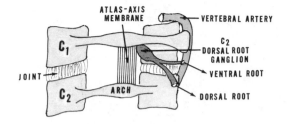

Figure 2–3. Greater superior occipital nerve emergence. The C_2 dorsal ganglion lies under the obliquus inferior muscle (not shown) over the lateral atlantoaxial point. It is adherent upon the capsule with fascia. The C_2 nerve emerges lateral to the posterior atlas-axial membrane and does not penetrate it. It passes on laterally to divide into a dorsal and ventral root.

a bifurcation of these two muscles, and is held there in a sling termed Schultze's bundle (Fig. 2–5). In the lower cervical segment (C_3 to C_8) the sensory and motor branches merge to form the nerve root, which then enter the intervertebral foramen. There are no foramina in the upper cervical segment. This has been specifically described.

As the lower spinal nerve segments that form the roots enter the foramen (Fig. 2–6), the motor (ventral) root (see Fig. 2–1) of the nerve is in intimate contact with the joint of von Luschka, and the sensory (dorsal) root lies close to the articular processes and its joint capsule.

The cervical nerve root normally occupies only one-fifth to one-fourth of the foramen. It varies in its relationship to the foraminal walls, and it is protected from compression by its coverings and sheaths.

The combined nerve fibers, sensory and motor, are considered to be a root. Each root is assigned a number indicating its level of departure from the cervical spine and its ultimate distribution into the upper extremities.

Each root descends anteriorly and laterally into the intervertebral foramina (Fig. 2–7) contained within a dural sleeve (Fig. 2–8) which in turn contains fibers of segmental autonomic nerves, capillaries, venules, lymphatics, nervous nervosum fibers, and spinal fluid. The nerve roots continue through the foramen to emerge and to divide immediately into an anterior and posterior primary division.

The number designated for a specific root is associated with the vertebra forming the intervertebral foramina. Essentially each nerve root emerges from a specific cervical vertebral level (Fig. 2–9). Enumeration of specific intervertebral disks is useful clinically. Inasmuch as there are not disks at every cervical level, this latter designation remains ambiguous.

There are no disks between the occiput, the atlas, and the axis. Anatomically there are no intervertebral foramina between these three cervical vertebrae. No numeric designation, therefore, is possible to relate these nerves in relationship to a disk level or foramen. They do have a relationship, however, to a specific vertebra.

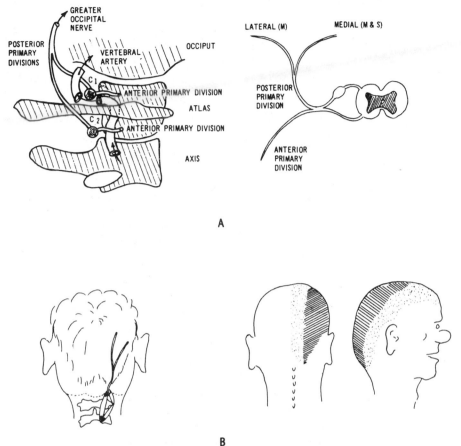

Figure 2–4. Upper cervical functional units (occipito-atlanto-axial). (A) The course of the C_1 and C_2 nerves as they merge into the occipital nerve and their relationship to the vertebral artery in the atlas-axis region. (B) Area (shaded) of hypesthesia, hyperesthesia, or anesthesia in the scalp area from pressure or irritation of these nerve roots.

The relationship of the dura to the nerve roots plays such a vital role in normal function and in pathologic symptomatology that it merits special emphasis.

The nerve root enters the foramen contained within its individual dural sheath. The dura lines the entire cord within the spinal canal of the cervical vertebral column. At each segmental level in the cord numerous fila emerge from the cord and merge into a root. The dorsal roots arise in the dorsal column of the cord, and the motor roots arise from the anterior horn cells of the cord (see Fig. 2–2).

At each level the fila merging into specific roots invaginate the dural and bring a *sleeve* with the nerve root into the foramen (Fig. 2–10). The layers that line the nerve roots are depicted in Figure 2–11 as follows:

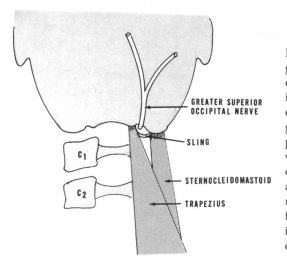

Figure 2–5. Occipital emergence of the greater superior occipital nerve. The greater occipital nerve (primarily C_2) emerges superficially at the groove medial to the mastoid process of the occiput. It leaves via an opening between the site of attachment of the trapezius and the sternocleidomastoid muscles upon the cranium. A fascial sling completes the opening through which the nerve emerges.

1. The *arachnoid lining* is located immediately adjacent to the nerve roots. It forms a subarachnoid cavity, which contains spinal fluid. The arachnoid terminates at the outer orifice of the intervertebral foramen.
2. The arachnoid forms a *septum* separating the sensory and motor components of the nerve roots within the foramen.
3. The *dural sheath* proceeds with the mixed nerve from the foramen into the peripheral nerve. This dura arachnoid covering continues with the nerve root as the *periradicular sheath* (Fig. 2–12).
4. There is a contained space outside the dura, termed the *epidural space*.
5. The *ligamentum flavum* is an elastin sheath that lines the inner aspect of the spinal canal and attaches to the capsule of the zygapophyseal joints (facets).

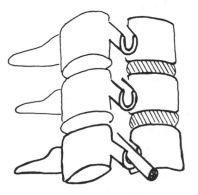
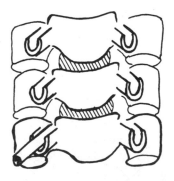

Figure 2–6. Direction of foraminal grooves: diagram depicting the downward-forward direction of the cervical nerve root.

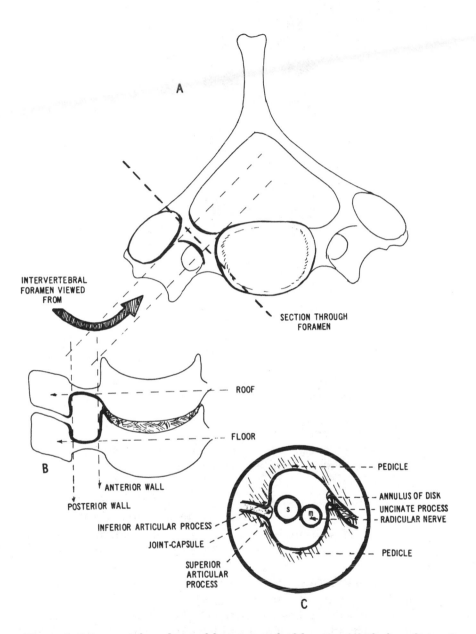

Figure 2–7. Anatomic boundaries of the intervertebral foramen. (A) The boundaries of
the foramen when viewed from the outside looking toward the spinal canal (large arrow)
reveal the walls, roof, and floor as depicted in (B). The mixed nerve (s=the sensory portion, m=the motor portion) in (C). The relationship of the sensory fibers to the posterior
articulations, and the relationship of the motor fibers to Luschka's joints and intervertebral disk are shown.

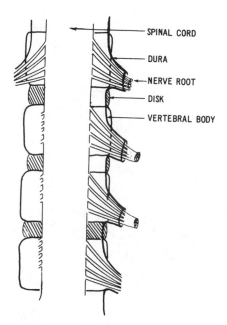

SPINAL CORD

DURA

NERVE ROOT

DISK

VERTEBRAL BODY

Figure 2–8. Formation and location of cervical nerve roots. The fila of the nerve roots emerge from the spinal cord at the level of the vertebral body, and the space between the group of fila that form the nerve roots is at the disk level. The relationship of nerve root to the disk is one of the reasons that disk herniation rarely impinges upon the nerve. The nerve root pierces the dura, and the dura.accompanies the nerve as a sleeve.

6. The *posterior longitudinal ligament*, which lines the posterior outer aspect of the disk annulus, continues distally to join the periradicular sheath.

Any or all of these tissues are capable of undergoing inflammation. Many are highly innervated so that they can become sites of nociceptive reaction.

The periradicular sheath becomes the epineural sheath of the brachial plexus (see Fig. 1–24). This sheath is firmly attached to the bony surfaces of the transverse process of the vertebrae and thus prevents the cord from being avulsed when there is excessive traction applied to the plexus. There are also attachments of this sheath to the scalene muscles.

The nerve root fila, as they emerge from the cord, face outward, anteriorly and downward into the internal orifice of the intervertebral foramina. As the foramina change in their configuration during flexion, extension, lateral flexion, and rotation of the head and neck, the relationship of the nerve roots within the canals varies. Both the foraminal openings and the nerve roots with their dural lining differ in configuration.

In forward flexion the cervical canal lengthens. The posterior wall elon-

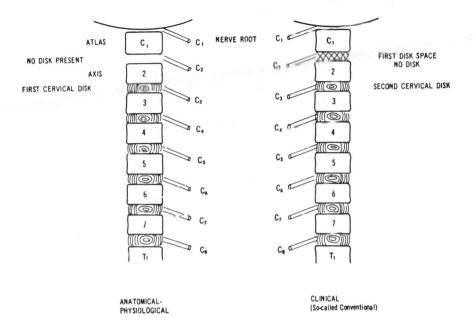

Figure 2–9. Nerve root location with regard to disk level.

gates more than does the anterior wall (Fig. 2–13). In extension the reverse occurs: The entire spinal canal shortens. The contents of the canal are thus subjected to dynamic changes in both length and width. The foramina also undergo
changes in size and configuration as the spine flexes and extends.

The cord within the spinal canal ascends and descends as the neck flexes
and extends. In flexion the cord elongates by virtue of its plasticity. The dura,
however, does not elongate, because it has little or no plasticity. The dura is plicated against the cord, with the plications being eliminated during elongation
of the cord (see Fig. 1–18).

Not only does the cord elongate, as does its dural sheath, but the nerve
roots that emerge at each spinal level also change in their angulation of emergence (Fig. 2–14). Normally the nerve roots formed from a grouping of fila from
the cord emerge at a downward and slightly anterior angle. They proceed therefrom into the foramina, and then laterally and anteriorly down the foraminal
gutter.

The dural sleeves of the nerve roots are also plicated. They are taut when
elongated and flexed when relaxed. When the neck is flexed, the cord has been
elongated and the nerve roots become more acutely angled as their emergence
from the cord moves cephalad (Fig. 2–14). The nerve roots and their dural
sheaths elongate, and the sheath thus becomes implicated

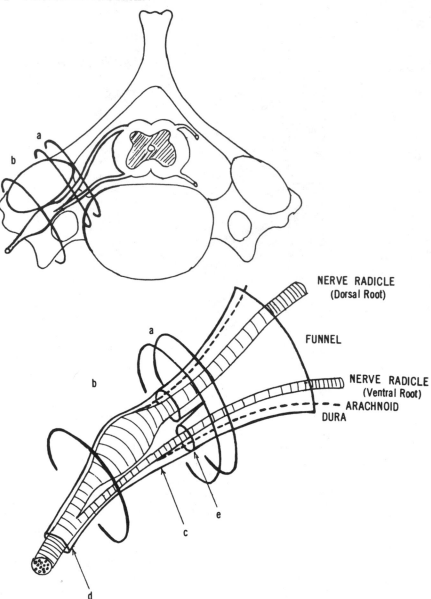

Figure 2–10. Dura-arachnoid sleeve of nerve root in the intervertebral canal.

a = intervertebral foramen
b = gutter of the transverse process
c = at this point the arachnoid attaches to the dura and prevents spinal fluid from going further
d = nerve from here on has only a dural coating
e = at apex of funnel, due to the inter-radicula septum, there are two ostia, one for the sensory and one for the motor roots

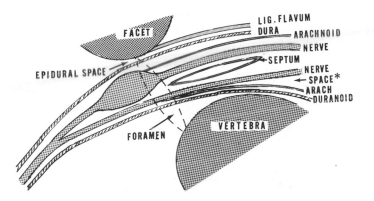

Figure 2–11. Schematic cross-section of contents of intervertebral foramen depicts the layers of tissues lining the nerve roots as they emerge from the cord and enter the spinal canal. The ligamentum flavum lines the posterior inner wall of the spinal canal and ends at the facet area. The dura continues with the nerve root into the extraspinal region. The arachnoid space (°) contains spinal fluid which terminates at the orifice of the foramen.

If the foramina through which the nerve roots emerge were not changed—that is, were also elongated in shape and size—a sharp angulation of the nerve would occur at the proximal orifice of the foramen. Compression of the nerve root would occur at the bony circumference of the foramen.

The nerve root canals (foramina) open (elongate) during spinal flexion, which allows more room for the emerging nerve root (see Fig. 1–16).

THE SYMPATHETIC NERVOUS SYSTEM

There are two major components of the sympathetic nervous system affecting the cervical spine region. Both components are involved in the circulatory, sweat gland, and hair follicle effects, but how they relate to pain from and in the cervical region remains controversial.

The two components are the *sympathetic chain* and the *vertebral nerve*. The cervical spinal cord does not contain intermediolateral horn cells from which preganglionic fibers arise. The preganglionic fibers in the neck arise from the thoracic cord intermediolateral horn cells and ascend to the cervical ganglia (Fig. 2–15).

All cervical nerve rami are gray, unmyelinated postganglionic nerves which have originated at synapses in the ganglia, with the preganglionic fibers from the thoracic spine. These gray rami proceed in three directions:

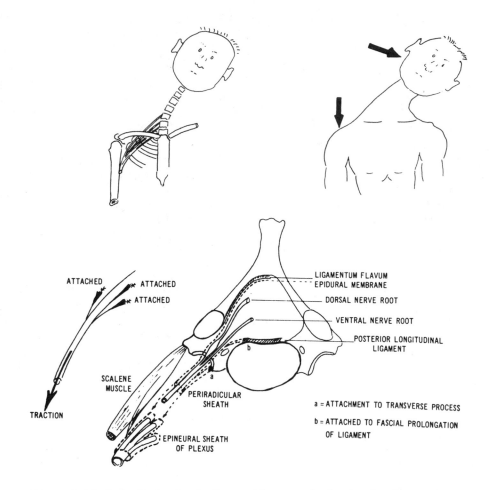

Figure 2–12. Periradicular sheath of nerve. The periradicular sheath is loose and becomes adherent at the plexus level. The scalene muscles have points of attachment to the brachial plexus.

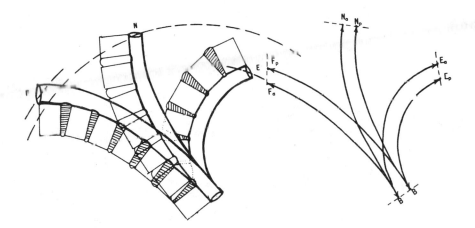

Figure 2–13. Alteration in spinal canal length. Length of neutral (N) spinal canal compared with that in flexion (F) and extension (E). In flexion the canal is longer and the anterior wall (Fa–B) is shorter than the posterior wall (Fa–B). In extension the total length of the canal is shorter, with the anterior (Ea–B) longer than the posterior wall (Ea–B). In neutral position both walls of the canal (Na–B and Na–B) are equal.

1. They accompany the nerve roots into the anterior and posterior primary rami to their destiny (sensory and motor) in the posterior cervical tissues and the upper extremities (extraforaminal).
2. They synapse with postganglionic fibers that proceed to the eyes, cranial nerves, arteries of the head and neck, and to the cardiac plexus (extraforaminal).
3. They accompany a sensory branch of the spinal nerve root to form the *sinuvertebral nerve* (Luschka's nerve or recurrent meningeal nerve) to return through the intervertebral foramen into the spinal canal. This nerve is considered to be the sensory nerve to the dura, the posterior longitudinal ligament, and the outer annular disk fibers (intraforaminal).

The vertebral nerve is a vasomotor nerve to the artery that runs through the vertebral foramina of the transverse processes of the vertebral bodies (Fig. 2–16).

Whether nociperception is transmitted via the sympathetic chain or the vertebral artery nerve is a matter of controversy. It is a well-accepted fact that pain or paresthesia is transmitted via sympathetic nerves. Pain in the face, cranial nerve distribution, and skull are attributed to irritation of the sympathetic nerve supply to these tissues. The Barré-Lieou syndrome has been attributed to irritation of the vertebral nerve, and symptoms consist of vertigo, facial pain, headache, tinnitus, nasal disturbance, facial flushing, and pharyngeal paresthesia.

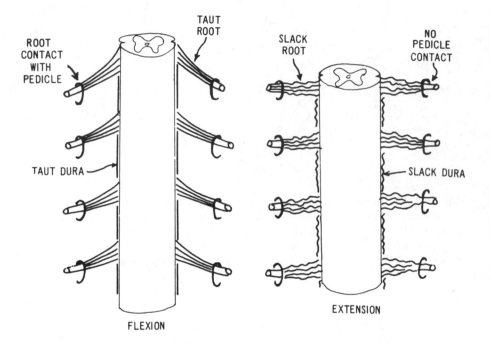

Figure 2–14. Relationship of nerve root within foramen during neck movement. During neck flexion (ventroflexion) the dura of the cord is pulled taut in physiologic tension, and the nerve roots emerging from the lateral sulcus of the cord are also under tension. The nerve roots appear to ascend, but they merely become taut and occupy the upper portion of the foramen and contact the under border of the pedicle above. In the extended position the dura pleat, as do the nerve roots; so the nerve is now slack, broader, but central in the foramen and away from the pedicle border.

Clinically, when the sympathetic nerve component is considered as a causative factor in the production of symptoms, a stellate block has been undertaken, often with benefit. Beta-adrenergic blocking agents have also been valuable, as have contrast moist applications: ice alternating with heat. These are all clinical judgments with an as yet unproven neurophysiologic basis.

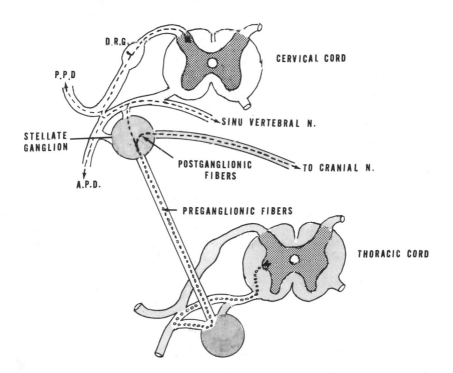

Figure 2–15. Sympathetic nervous system.

The preganglionic (white) fibers originate from the intermediolateral horn cells of the thoracic cord and ascend to the stellate ganglion where they synapse with the postganglionic gray fibers. All the extravertebral fibers of the cervical spine are gray.

The gray fibers form the recurrent meningeal nerve (sinovertebral nerve of Luschka) to innervate the dura, the outer annular fibers, and the posterior longitudinal ligament.

There is branching to the salivary glands, cranial nerve, and the dilators of the pupil. There is innervation to the arteries to the head and neck, the cardiac plexus, and the subclavian brachial plexus.

There are sympathetic fibers that accompany the somatic nerves in the posterior primary division (PPDP) and the anterior primary division (APD). The sensory fibers emanate from the dorsal root ganglia (DRG).

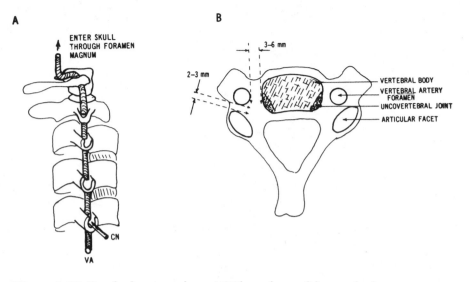

Figure 2–16. Vertebral artery pathway. (*A*) The pathway of the vertebral artery as it ascends through the foramina. (*B*) The relationship of the foramen to the vertebral body, the uncovertebral Luschka joint, and the zygapophyseal (facet) joint is evident. The space difference between body and foramen (3–6 mm) and facet foramen (2–3 mm) indicate that vascular impingement is most commonly due to encroachment by the superior articular process and rarely due to changes of the uncovertebral joints.

REFERENCES

Bogduk, N: The clinical anatomy of the cervical dorsal root. Spine 7:4, 1982.
Hunter, CR and Mayfield, FH: Role of the upper cervical roots in the production of pain in the head. Am J Surg 78:743, 1949.

BIBLIOGRAPHY

DePalma, AF and Rothman, RH: The Intervertebral Disc. WB Saunders, Philadelphia, 1970.
Fielding, JW: Cineroentgenography of the normal cervical spine. J Bone Joint Surg 39A:1280, 1957.
Gracvetsky, S: The Spinal Engine. Springer-Verlag, New York, 1988.
Hadley, LA: The Spine: Anatomico-radiographic Studies: Development and the Cervical Region. Charles C Thomas, Springfield, IL, 1956.
Herlihy, WF: Sinuvertebral nerve. New Zealand Medical Journal 48:214, 1949.
Jackson, R: The Cervical Syndrome, ed 2. Charles C Thomas, Springfield, IL, 1958.
Jones, MD: Cineradiographic studies of the normal cervical spine. California Medicine 93:293, 1960.

Orofino, C, Sherman, MS, and Schechter, D: Luschka's joints—a degenerative phenomenon. J Bone Joint Surg 42A:853, 1960.

Werne, S: The possibilities of movement in the craniovertebral joints. Acta Orthop Scand XXVIII: 165, 1959.

White, AA and Gordon, SL (eds): American Academy of Orthopedic Surgeons: Symposium on Idiopathic Low Back Pain. CV Mosby, St. Louis, 1982.

Wiesel, SW, Feffer, HL, and Rothman, RH: Neck Pain. Mitchie, Charlottesville, VA, 1986.

CHAPTER 3

Posture

Posture is the attitude the human being assumes upon standing or sitting in the erect position (Fig. 3–1). Posture has cosmetic application in "how we look." Posture has psychologic implication in that we stand the way we feel. Posture is influenced by familial and congenital factors, modified by training and habit, influenced by peer appearance, dictated by occupational demands, and adversely affected by illness of orthopedic or neurologic consequence.

Posture can also cause or influence numerous orthopedic and neurologic diseases or syndromes of pain and impairment. Faulty posture augments tissue changes in bony, ligamentous, and muscular structures and is thought to adversely affect the spinal column discogenic tissues. Therefore, it merits thorough evaluation.

CHRONOLOGIC DEVELOPMENT OF POSTURE

The spine of the newborn infant, yet to react to gravity and to assume an erect position, has none of the adult physiologic curves. The entire newborn spine retains the *in utero* posture, which is that of total flexion (kyphosis). The curvature of the newborn spine forms a slightly greater kyphotic curve than the physiologic kyphotic curve of the thoracic spine which will remain throughout life.

The newborn spine has no lordotic curves, neither in the cervical area nor in the lumbar area (Fig. 3–2). The first lordotic curve of the vertebral column is noted in the cervical region during the first six or eight weeks of life. At this stage of development the newborn child extends his or her head from the prone position. This head-neck extension is an antigravity action which occurs by virtue of contraction of the extensor muscles. The action occurs with some

43

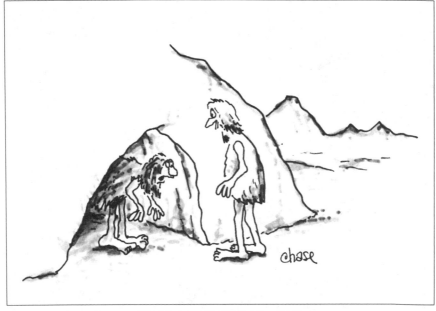

"I tried standing erect, but I kept banging my head!"

Figure 3–1. Comic spoof of erect posture.
(From John Chase, reprinted from Science 43:17, March, 1989, with permission of the artist.)

proprioceptive input and initiation from the basic righting reflexes.

The ultimate cervical lordotic curve remains throughout the life of the individual, with daily variations from change of position and various activities. The cervical spine is flexible and adheres to the laws of gravity and to muscular action imparted to it. There are numerous factors that modify the degree of curvature of the cervical spine, and they will be discussed here.

Because the cervical spine is the uppermost curve and supports the head, it is dependent on the lower spinal column curves: the thoracic, lumbar, and sacral curves.

All the superincumbent curves are flexible and depend upon ligamentous and capsular support and muscular tone to remain erect. The muscular tone is the predominant—but not the only—source of support and is the major factor that determines the degrees of spinal curvatures in their relationship to the center of gravity.

NEUROLOGIC CONCEPTS OF POSTURE

The degree of muscular tone is dependent upon proprioceptive feedback from the periphery. Proprioceptive impulses ascend from the ground upward

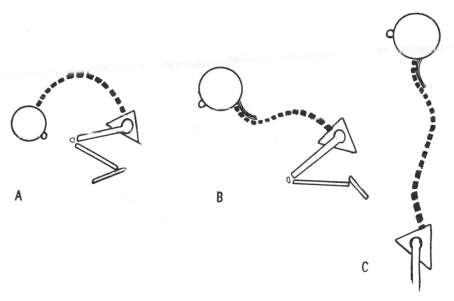

Figure 3–2. Chronologic development of cervical lordosis in the development of posture. (A) The curve of the fetal spine *in utero*. (B) Formation of the cervical lordosis when the head overcomes gravity. (C) Erect adult posture.

through the central nervous system to inform the body of its relationship to the center of gravity (Fig. 3–3).

The proprioceptive *end organs* are located within the skin, the joint capsules, the ligaments, and the muscles of the entire body and are stimulated by pressure variants, movements, and peripheral sensations of touch. In its contact with the ground, the foot receives sensory contact through the skin, the muscles, the bones, the ligaments, the joints, and the capsules. There are similar sensations received from the ankles, the knees, the hips, the pelvis, and on up the spine. All proprioceptive fibers from these end organs send instantaneous information which becomes coordinated in the central nervous system to initiate appropriate muscular tone.

The vestibular system also sends information to the central nervous system to inform the body of its relationship to the center of gravity. These righting reflexes are inherent in the central nervous system at birth and are modified during development as the external and internal situations change.

It becomes apparent that the sensation, considered proprioceptive here, is instrumental in maintaining the erect posture and that it influences the relationship of the erect body to the center of gravity. The sensation also is impressed upon the cortex, which interprets the sensation of the total erect person.

The sensory motor nervous system thus is the major determinant in the

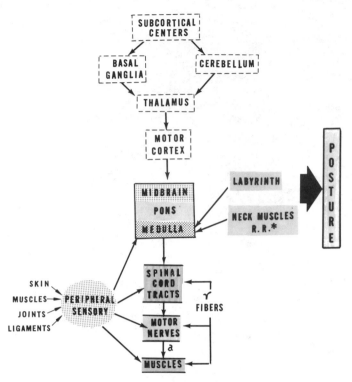

Figure 3–3. Neurologic concept of posture. The upper neurologic pathways (subcortical centers, basal ganglia, cerebellum, thalamus, and motor cortex) are the well-documented circuits by which motor activities are initiated and coordinated.

Within the midbrain medulla are the primary righting reflex centers that receive impulses from the labyrinth and the righting reflexes (°R.R.) of the neck muscles. Posture is dependent upon this medullary center and the spinal cord interneurons influencing the motor nerves that are moderated by the alpha and gamma fibers to the muscles.

Each level of the central system receives and is moderated by peripheral sensory impulses from the skin, joints, capsules, ligaments, and muscles (see text).

process of assuming the erect posture. Because the erect posture is also that of superincumbent curves as they relate to the center of gravity, the degrees of curves are solely dependent upon proprioception. The curves are also influenced by appropriate perception of the erect position. Posture is, therefore, a reflex proprioceptive mechanism that depends upon cortical appreciation and acceptance.

It should be apparent now that posture is a neuromuscular reaction to proprioceptive impulses from the periphery and that the *feeling* of that posture as normal or abnormal is a learned process.

Further on in the individual's maturation, the thoracic curve becomes less flexible to the extent that there is no further significant flexion or extension in sagittal motion of the total spine. The thoracic spine of an adult person is essentially fixed in its kyphosis. The spinal curves above and below this dorsal kyphosis must, therefore, be correlated in maintaining the erect posture in its relationship to the center of gravity. An increase in the lumbar lordosis accentuates the cervical lordosis, and vice versa.

DEVELOPMENTAL CONCEPTS OF POSTURE

Admittedly the ultimate spinal curves are initially determined by developmental factors related to gravity. These curves form the erect posture. As a person develops there are at least three major factors that influence adult posture: heredity, disease, and acquired habit. Of the three, the last is the least well-understood. However, it is the factor that can be influenced most by treatment.

The familial-hereditary factors influencing the posture of the adult patient can be discerned by evaluation of the parents, grandparents, and/or siblings. This familial posture is essentially a body type and may be altered slightly, but it is more difficult to modify than that which is acquired.

Disease factors influencing posture are too numerous to discuss fully here. Examples include inflammatory joint disease (such as rheumatoid spondylitis), other rheumatoid disease, neurologic diseases (such as parkinsonism), and the effects of structural scoliosis. There are many others that can be detected in the patient's history by careful examination and through x-ray confirmation. Aspects of faulty posture resulting from disease can be modified during the development of the disease if its impact on the posture is recognized.

THE FEELING OF PROPER POSTURE—DEVELOPMENTAL CONCEPT

The posture of acquired habit has been considered a neuromuscular phenomenon that has its inception in early childhood. Many factors affecting the growing child play a role in this concept (Feldenkrais).

The feeling of proper erect posture develops as the nervous patterns develop. From the ground up there is proprioception ascending to the neck. The head assumes a normal balance upon the neck when there is comfort and ease in remaining erect. All proprioception is subconscious, yet it constantly bombards the righting reflexes to maintain erect posture.

There is little or no need to be aware of all the components of the body involved in the erect posture. When all proprioception influencing the muscles of the erect spine results in the person feeling that his or her posture is *normal*, the posture is correct, effortless, cosmetically proper, and pain-free.

The erect stance and body position *feels* like a *proper* posture. The vestibular apparatus within the head also imparts proprioception which, when considered to be a proper posture by the *feeling*, asserts no effort to modify the righting reflexes.

Whatever modifies or influences the resultant reflex action gives the feeling of *normal* or *correct* posture. What are some of these factors which lay down the neuromuscular patterns? What influences the proprioceptions? More important what remains when the pattern is considered normal by *feel* yet is structurally faulty or abnormal.

Postural bad habits develop in childhood. The slumped-over posture is seen often in adolescents and young adults. The posture assumed becomes so habitual that it becomes normal—it feels normal. Slumped posture may be the result of family or peer pressure: the result of anxiety, insecurity, fear, anger or despondency in childhood. Daily activities may influence posture. Feldenkrais suggests that many postures develop from the "cringing from fear of physical assault by domineering parents or siblings."

Over the years, the assumed posture becomes comfortable and accepted as normal. The proprioceptive stimuli of this assumed posture have no impact upon the cortical interpretation. The posture—for example, the forward head posture—is accepted, and the muscular tone needed to support this posture is also accepted (Fig. 3–4). The person perceives no need to correct the assumed posture because there is no discomfort or fatigue initially.

The fact is that the posture holding the head forward of the center of gravity is ignored (see Fig. 3–4) although it demands excessive muscular action.

Unconscious bad habits develop in adolescence. Self-consciousness in a person who feels too tall may cause a slumped-forward posture, or a young woman whose breasts are larger than those of her peers might hold her shoulders forward. The persistence of the assumed posture after many years becomes accepted as normal for that individual and continues into life long after the original cause. The pattern is now well-established not only in the neuromuscular complex, but also in the musculoskeletal system.

ACQUIRED POSTURAL INFLUENCES

The acquired posture is also influenced by daily activities that demand a forward head posture. Some jobs, such as operating a computer and viewing the screen, require a forward head posture. Faulty vision or correction by bifocal or trifocal glasses may place demands upon the posture that are undesirable. Causative factors such as these demand a careful study of the activities of daily living (ADL) to determine their effect upon the posture.

The emotions also influence posture. We stand, sit, and walk *as we feel*. The depressed person walks, stands, and sits in a depressed manner. The angry person projects tension in his or her stance. The impatient individual depicts im-

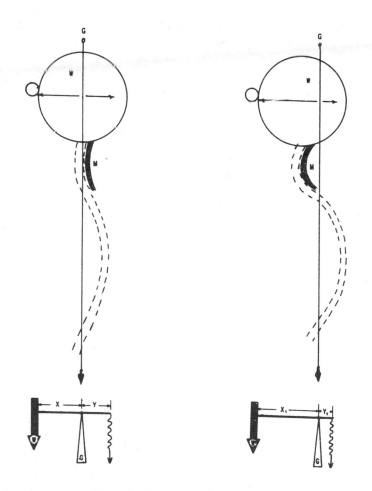

Figure 3–4. Gravity effect on a forward-head posture with increased lordosis.

W   =   weight of the head; remains constant.

X   =   distance of head weight (W) from center of gravity (G).

Y   =   distance of spinal musculature from center of gravity (G).

M   =   tension developed by musculature to sustain weight of head (W),

$$W \times X = M \times Y$$

In a simple lever system the weight supported by the fulcrum G is the sum of the weights acting at each end of the lever bar. Any change in the length of the lever bar must be compensated by a change in weight to maintain balance.

If W is 10 lbs, and distance X is 6 inches, the force exerted by M through lever arm Y of 4 inches is 15 lbs.

If lever arm X increases to 8 inches, a forward shift of 2 inches, the weight of the head remains constant, the posterior lever arm Y decreases to 2 inches, and muscle tension must increase to 40 pounds. This increase not only is fatiguing but also acts as a compressive force on the soft tissues, including the disk.

patience in posture as well as in actions. The subject of body language is now widely researched and is recognized by the astute practitioner. Its effect on undesirable posture must be recognized and addressed.

BIBLIOGRAPHY

Boyd, IA, et al: The role of the gamma system in movement and posture. Association for the Aid of Crippled Children, New York, 1964.

Brunnstrom, S: Clinical Kinesiology, ed. 3. FA Davis, Philadelphia, 1972.

Burke, D and Eklund, G: Muscle spindle activity in man during standing. Acta Physiol Scand 100:187, 1977.

Ertekin, N and Ertekin, C: Erector spinae muscle responses while standing. J Neurol Neurosurg Psychiatry 44:73, 1981.

Feldenkrais, M: Body and Mature Behavior. International University Press, New York, 1973.

Joseph, J: Man's Posture: Electromyographic Studies. Charles C Thomas, Springfield, IL, 1960.

Kelton, IW and Wright, RD: The mechanism of easy standing by man. Australian Journal of Experimental Biology and Medical Science 27:505, 1949.

Lovett, RW: Lateral curvature of the spine and round shoulders. P. Blakiston, Philadelphia, 1907.

Roaf, R: Posture. Academic Press, New York, 1977.

CHAPTER 4

Neck and Arm Pain: Tissue Sites and Mechanisms

To know the normal and to recognize deviation from normal; to understand the tissue responsible and to be able to reproduce the pain by reproducing specific motions and positions—this is the principle for diagnosing neck and arm pain. Nowhere in the human skeletal system is this principle more applicable than in pain and disability originating in or from the cervical spine.

Pain in and from the neck region is variously described and may originate from various tissue sites within the cervical spine. Pain also may be produced by numerous mechanisms through various pathways. Pain may be felt in various areas of the neck and in the upper extremities. With so many variables, how is it possible to simplify accurate diagnosis by applying the formula stated above?

The following discussion of pain and impairment from the cervical spine will relate exclusively to *benign* pain syndromes and not to pain and impairment from fracture, metabolic disease, malignancies or other organic disease entities. True pathology occurs in these benign problems, and these organic components will be discussed.

The gross structural and functional anatomy has been reviewed. The nervous system, which carries sensations from various tissues, has been delineated. It remains to be clarified as to which tissue(s) can become the site(s) of pain. It must be ascertained which movement or position caused or causes the claimed pain or impairment. Clarification of the tissue responsible and the movement or position implemented forms the basis for appropriate treatment.

Recent studies have elucidated which tissues within the cervical spine, when irritated or inflamed, are capable of eliciting pain. The tissue reaction causing the production of nociceptive agents that affect the end organs of the sensory nerves with resultant pain is becoming more evident. Production of nociceptor agents, however, must affect the end organs of nerves located in specific tissues capable of transmission of pain sensations. These nocioceptive elements will be discussed further, but first the tissue site within the cervical spine must be specified (Fig. 4–1).

The cervical disk became the *bête noire* of cervical pain when the intervertebral disk was identified as *the* site of pain in the functional units of the vertebral spinal column. That the disk plays a major role in the production of pain and disability is accepted, and it does so to a significant degree; chapter 7 is devoted to this subject.

Cloward attempted to clarify the exact role of pain originating within the intervertebral disk. He injected dye into the nucleus in an attempt to produce a *diskogram*. By injecting dye, not only would the configuration of the disk be clarified, but the precise pain resulting from a specific disk would be designated.

In performing the diskogram Cloward ascertained that the anterior longitudinal ligament was sensitive. Upon touching the ligament with the needle of the diskogram, a pain was elicited that the awake patient localized in both site and type of pain. Cloward assumed that the tissue he was touching with the diskogram needle was the outer layer of the disk annulus. He thereupon desig-

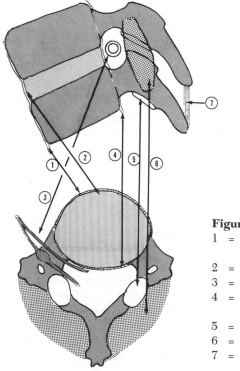

Figure 4–1. Nociceptor sites:

1 = anterior longitudinal ligament
2 = outer annulus
3 = dura
4 = posterior longitudinal ligament
5 = facet capsule
6 = muscle
7 = ligaments

nated the mechanism as *diskogenic* pain versus *neurogenic* pain when the nerve roots within the foramina are involved (Fig. 4–2). The sites of projection from diskogenic pain were at the paraspinous sites at thoracic level with each cervical spine level radiating to a precise level (Cloward). This radiation was not a dermatomic area, inasmuch as there could be no nerve root involved in an anterior approach injection. The referred area was assumed to be a *sclerotome* area. The anterior longitudinal ligament considered to be the nociceptive site is innervated by the sinu vertebral nerve.

The posterior longitudinal ligament is also known to be innervated by the recurrent sinu vertebral nerve and is considered to be a site of nociception. A common, if not the sole manner, in which the posterior longitudinal ligament can be involved in pain production is by encroachment from the central posterior protruding annular layers of the intervertebral disk.

In Cloward's classic paper, the midline posterior disk protrusion implicated this protrusion "from the four lower cervical disks to refer pain to the midline posteriorly in the back of the neck and upper shoulder." He implied that the sensory nerves responsible for this pain included the anterior and posterior longitudinal ligaments and the peripheral annular fiber layers. Similar studies in the lumbar spine (Falconer, et al), implicated the posterior longitudinal ligament. Thus the same tissue site in the cervical spine can be implicated.

The nerve roots are a tissue site of nociception, but the exact site within the nerve complex and the mechanism of irritation remains equivocal. The nerve roots per se are not considered the site for referred pain. Pressure upon a nerve anywhere in the body is not a primary cause of pain. Pressure upon nerves may cause paresthesia and ultimately hypalgesia and hypesthesia with subsequent anesthesia and motor paresis—not principally pain. What allows the nerve root within the foramen to emit pain when compressed?

The dura is now considered to be the site of pain production. The dura is innervated by the sinuvertebral nerve. The mechanism by which the dura is implicated is that of traction or compression wherein the enclosed nerve roots are rendered ischemic. Within the dural sheath are contained capillaries, venules, lymphatics, and the nervi nervorum fibers. Ischemia or mechanical pressure of these enclosed tissues can result in pain (Hoyland, et al). The benefit derived from epidural injection of an anesthetic and a steroid indicates that pain must occur from irritation of these tissues.

The nerve roots within the dural sheath are motor, somatosensory, and sympathetic. Testing of nerve reaction (Frykholm) indicated the sensory nerve root as a prominent site of pain production *in a dermatomic distribution*. Stimulation of the ventral (motor) fiber caused a deep, boring, unpleasant sensation in a sclerotomal region without necessarily causing a muscular contraction. It thus appears that the response is sensory phenomenon, not from a forceful painful muscular contraction. It must be noted, however, that the sensation is noted in the region of the muscle group innervated by the specific ventral nerve root.

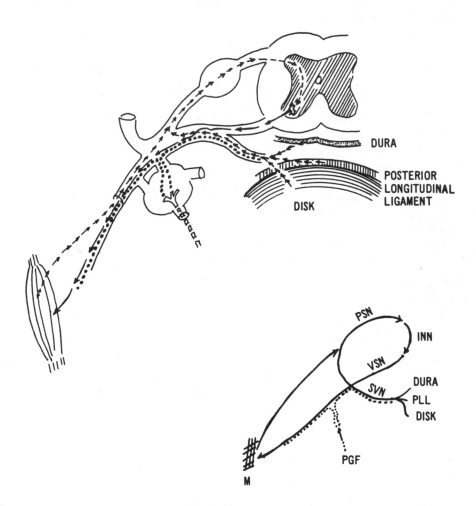

Figure 4–2. Postulated mechanism of disk pain (sciatica or brachialgia). The sinuverte-bral nerve (SVN) originating or located in the annulus fibrosus (disk), in the longitudinal ligaments (PLL), or in the dura mater (dura) enters the main nerve trunk and runs along the posterior spinal nerve (PSN). The arc to the anterior horn cell is via the internuncial nerve (INN), and the impulses leave along the ventral motor root (VSN) to the muscle (M), causing painful muscle spasm. This *myalgic* or sclerotomic pain returns via the sen-sory pathway back to the sensory root (PSN). As depicted in the lower half of this figure, the sympathetic postganglionic fibers (PGF) accompany the sinuvertebral nerve (SVN) and the anterior primary ramus to the muscle.

It behooves us to analyze the chemical influences upon the nociceptors that, in addition to mechanical factors, result in the transmission of pain. Endogenously occurring chemical substances that have an excitatory effect upon the nociceptors are hydrogen ions, serotonin, histamine, bradykinin, and prostaglandins. A well-documented cycle of chemical nociceptor irritation is the sequela of the breakdown of phospholipids into arachidonic acid into prostaglindin E. Corticosteroids are known to intervene in the breakdown of phospholipids into arachidonic acid, thus accounting for their anti-inflammatory action. Acetylsalicylic acid (aspirin) also inhibits arachidonic acid breakdown to prostaglandin E.

Prostaglandin E excites the nerve endings. Bradykinin affects the blood vessels, causing dilatation and increased permeability with release of substance P, which becomes an excitor of the end organs of the nerves. Mechanically there is also the effect of heat or ice upon the nerve endings (Bromm).

The nerve roots also have been studied in regard to transmission of various sensation. Pain is mediated via the dorsal roots after they have been distally activated at their end organs. The unmyelinated nerves transmit the sensation ultimately interpreted as pain. There is also a portion (25 percent) of the motor nerves that are sensory, and stimulation or irritation of one of these motor nerves can result in pain. This mechanism is considered the basis for the transmission of *sclerotomal* rather than *dermatomal* referred pain.

The flaval ligaments, which have the role of insuring that the facet capsules are not impinged in neck movement, are not innervated and thus have no nociceptive properties. The interspinous ligaments are undoubtedly innervated and may be a source of pain production but, other than the classic work of Kellgren, there are no precise studies on the nociceptive qualities of these ligaments.

Proceeding posteriorly in the cervical spine functional unit in quest of nociceptor sites we find the zygapophyseal (facet) joints to be definitely a source of pain. Bogduk emphasized the facet joints as the *source* rather than the *cause* of neck pain, but when the joints were locally anesthetized, the pain was relieved for the duration of the anesthetic agent. The facet joints are innervated by somatosympathetic fibers of the posterior primary division of the nerve root.

There are ultimate degenerative changes in the cartilage of facet joints, termed *arthritis*, but as a rule these changes are asymptomatic until trauma occurs; then it is probably the capsule that becomes the site of nociperception. As will be discussed in the section dealing with degenerative spondylosis, osteophytic changes can impinge upon the emerging nerve root through the intervertebral foramina.

The neck muscles, as muscles throughout the body, are also a site of nociperception. The anterior neck flexor muscles, implicated in acceleration injuries such as whiplash (see chapter 5) (Krout and Anderson), are a source of pain, as are the extensor (erector spinae) muscles.

Trauma to muscles termed *strain* or *sprain* are common and vary from mere elongation with resultant edema to microscopic or macroscopic hemorrhage (Malone and Garrett). A forceful muscular contraction may also cause trauma at the myofascial periosteal juncture with resultant pain and tenderness (Fig. 4–3).

Sustained muscular tension is also known to cause a mechanical vascular type of pain. Sustained isometric muscular contraction in an extremity, with and without a tourniquet applied to occlude arterial flow, has been well-documented as the cause of ischemic muscular pain. Sustained muscular isometric contraction has also been thoroughly studied (Travell and Simons) and termed *myofascial pain*. The mechanism of this pain has been postulated to be anxious, postural, occupational, and microscopic traumatic. Sustained muscular contraction

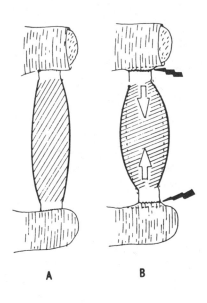
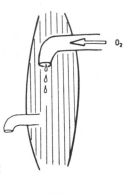
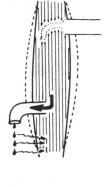

Figure 4–3. Pain production from myofascial-periosteal strain and muscle ischemia. (*A*) Relaxed muscle with no traction upon its myofascial-periosteal attachment. (*B*) The muscle contracted (shortened) with resultant traction stress upon the sensitive periosteum, causing pain and tenderness. (*C*) Inflow of nutritive blood (O_2) into a relaxed muscle not forming waste products, mp. (*D*) In the contracted muscle the source of oxygen is shut off, but the muscle is working and creating metabolic products irritating to muscle tissues. If the condition of (*D*) does not return to that of (*C*) and permit new blood to wash away *mp* and replenish the O_2 supply, the irritating mp cause pain.

accumulates excessive muscular metabolites, which become irritants and cause resultant muscular contraction. The contracted muscles literally constrict the intrinsic blood vessels, so that while there is excessive muscular contraction requiring blood supply there is diminished blood flow. Ischemia results, and there is venous lymphatic compression, which prevents *washing out* of the accumulated metabolites. A viscious circle results, with ischemic pain as the end point. All these are factors in the mechanisms of cervical muscular pain.

BIBLIOGRAPHY

Anrep, GV and Von Saalfeld, E: Blood flow through skeletal muscle in relation to its contraction. J Physiol 85:375, 1935.

Baetjer, AM: The diffusion of potassium from resting skeletal muscle following reduction in blood supply. Am J Physiol 112:139, 1935.

Barcroft, H and Millen, JLE: The blood-flow through muscle during sustained contraction. J Physiol 97:17, 1939.

Barcroft, H and Dornshurst, AC: The blood-flow through human calf during rhythmic exercise. J Physiol 109:402, 1949.

Bogduk, N and Marsland, A: The cervical zygapophyseal joints as a source of neck pain. Spine 13(6):610, 1988.

Bromm, B (ed): Pain measurement in man: Neurophysiological correlates of pain. Elsevier, New York, 1984.

Cloward, RB: Cervical diskography. Ann Surg 150(6):1052, 1959.

deVries, HA: Quantitative electromyographic investigation of the spasm theory of muscle pain. Am J Phys Med 45:119, 1966.

Dorpat, TL and Holmes, TH: Mechanisms of skeletal muscle pain and fatigue. AMA Archives of Neurology and Psychiatry. 74:528, 1955.

Falconer, MA, et al: Observations on cause and mechanism of symptom-production in sciatica and low-back pain. J Neurol Neurosurg Psychiatry 11:26, 1948.

Frykholm, R: Cervical nerve root compression resulting from disk degeneration and root sleeve fibrosis. Acta Chir Scand (Suppl 160) 1951.

Herlihy, WF: Sinu-vertebral nerve. New Zealand Med J 48:214, 1949.

Hill, AV: The pressure developed in muscle during contraction. J Physiol 107:518, 1948.

Hoyland, JA, Freemont, AJ, and Jayson, MIV: Intervertebral foramen venous obstruction: A cause of periradicular fibrosis. Spine 14:6, 1989.

Inman, VT and Saunders, JB de CM: Referred pain from skeletal structures. J Nerv Ment Dis 99:660, 1944.

Katz, LN, Lindner, E, and Landt, H: On the nature of the substances producing pain in the contracting skeletal muscle: Its bearing on the problems of angina pectoris and intermittent claudication. J Clin Invest 14:807, 1935.

Kellgren, JH: The anatomical source of back pain. Rheumatol Rehab 16:3-12, 1977.

Krout, RM and Anderson, TP: Role of anterior cervical muscles in production of neck pain. Arch Phys Med Rehab 47:603, 1966.

Malone, TR and Garrett, WE: Muscle strains: Histology, cause and treatment. Surgical Rounds for Orthopedics 43, Jan. 1989.

Neufeld, I: Mechanical factors in the pathogenesis, prophylaxis and management of fibrositis (fibropathic syndromes). Arch Phys Med Rehab 36:759, 1955.

Nikolaou, PK, et al: Biomechanical and histological evaluation of muscle after control strain injury. Am J Sports Med 15:9, 1987.

Orolino, C, Sherman, MS, and Schechter, D: Luschka's joint: A degenerative phenomenon. J Bone Joint Surg 42-A:853, 1960.

Perlow, S, Markle, P, and Katz, LN: Factors involved in the production of skeletal muscle pain. Arch Int Med 53:814, 1934.

Reed, JD: Effects of flexion-extension movements of the head and spine upon the spinal cord and nerve roots. J Neurol Neurosurg Psychiatry 23:214, 1960.

Sarno, JE: Etiology of neck and back pain: An autonomic myoneuralgia. J Nerv Ment Dis 169:55, 1981.

Steindler, A: The cervical pain syndrome.. In Edwards, JW (ed): Instructional Course Lectures. The American Academy of Orthopedic Surgeons, vol XIV. Ann Arbor, 1957.

Travell, JG and Simons, DG: Myofascial Pain and Dysfunction: The Trigger Point Manual. Williams & Wilkins, Baltimore, 1983.

Walton, JN: Disorders of Voluntary Muscle. Churchill Livingstone, London, 1974.

Weiberg, G: Back pain in relation to the nerve supply of the intervertebral disk. *Sweden.* Acta Orthop Scand 19:213, 1941.

CHAPTER 5

Mechanisms of Pain in the Neck and from the Neck

The tissue sites within the cervical spine and functional units capable of being nociceptor sites have been enumerated. To implement the principle as stated in chapter 2, "To know the normal and to recognize deviation from normal; . . . to be able to reproduce *the* pain by reproducing specific motions and positions," the mechanisms causing pain must be considered.

The two major causes of pain are *trauma* and *arthritis*. These terms need evaluation and verification. *Trauma* can be categorized into (1) external trauma, (2) posture, and (3) tension. *Arthritis* can be divided into (1) degenerative and (2) all the sequelae of acute inflammation.

TRAUMA

Trauma implies an external force which, to be detrimental and to cause symptoms, must initiate tissue changes within the cervical spine that exceed the normal movement or position of segments of the cervical spine. The elasticity or plasticity of the involved tissues must have been exceeded and/or traumatized to release nociceptor chemical substances.

Predominant in the concept of trauma are the external forces generated with subsequent tissue changes of the hyperflexion hyperextension injuries. This is a complex topic that will be given a full chapter discussion (chapter 6).

The mechanisms that injure tissues are ligamentous, capsular, muscular, diskogenic, and even neurologic. The history implicates the mechanism, and the examination verifies the residual tissue response. The normal flexion, extension, rotation, and lateral flexion range of motion have, as a rule, been exceeded. The ligaments and muscles, with their fascial compartments, have been moved in excess of normal physiologic range.

Subluxation is an appropriate term meaning that a minor portion of *luxation (dislocation)* has occurred. The normal constraining tissues normally are ligaments, muscles, their fascial containers, joint capsules, and even the annular disk fibers. Subluxation implies that these tissues have exceeded their restrictive function: Tissues have been damaged.

The history reveals the significance of the impact as to force, direction, experienced immediate reaction, and subsequent residual sensation. The preceding tissue condition of the injured individual can also indicate the potential damage incurred by these conditioned or deconditioned tissues from the external trauma.

Because range of motion is a criterion of the normalcy of the involved joint tissues and their periarticular tissues, this range must be tested. Knowledge of normal range of motion is the criterion against which to measure the current range. It must be remembered that each segment of the cervical spine has a specific direction and range of motion: flexion extension 35 degrees between occiput and atlas: rotation 80 to 90 degrees between atlas and axis: and combination of flexion, extension, rotation, and lateral flexion between each segment of the lower cervical spine.

The carefully performed examination depicts restriction at each of these segments. Pain and restriction at the end points of motion reveal the deviation from normal and at which specific cervical level. Limitation with or without pain implicates joint capsular tissues, ligaments, or myofascial muscular tissues.

Pain usually causes reflex muscular isometric contraction to *splint* the offended joint that has been traumatized. The muscular contraction, termed *protective spasm,* is a neuromuscular reflex. Its presence is manifested by guarding and thus limited motion. There is a feel noted by the examiner that reveals the difference between ligamentous articular limitation and the limitation of muscular guarding spasm. Range limitation is more segmental than general in articular-ligamentous involvement than it is in spasm. Tenderness is also more generalized in spasm. Spasm has the tendency to give slowly, although with limitation, upon gentle passive motion. Segmental limitation rather than general limitation indicates articular ligamentous restriction rather than muscular guarding.

Range of motion testing must be considered in the context of *passive* and *active*. *Passive* is the range of motion illicited by the examiner; *active* is the range of motion illicited by the patient. The former gives objective evaluation although restricted or influenced by the ability of the patient to be examined. Pain and fear will obviously influence the end result. Active range of motion is significantly more influenced by fear and pain tolerance.

Which soft tissue is involved—ligament, capsular, muscular, fascial, or even diskogenic—cannot be differentiated by the examiner inasmuch as all may play a part in the restriction and production of pain. There is a difference in the significance of tissue injury, however, that makes this differentiation less meaning-ful. Soft tissue injury—ligamentous, capsular, fascial, and muscular—has a less ominous future disabling result. Diskogenic damage with or without neurologic injury has a greater significance.

In performing and evaluating the examination, there is also the matter of the acuteness of the injury. The reaction immediately after injury, reaction within hours and/or days after the injury, and reaction after a longer time play a role in evaluation of the patient and his or her tissue reaction. In the initial immediate examination a state of shock may occur, with a variable emotional reaction. Ultimately this shock subsides and the incidental factors of emotional reaction blend and influence the reaction of the injured person. Fear, apprehension, anxiety, and even anger become involved, and any of these factors influences both passive and active evaluations of the person. These factors must be taken into consideration in documenting the results of the examination.

The differentiation between tissue damage and diskogenic and/or neurogenic damage will be fully discussed in the chapters on the cervical disk (chapter 7) and the whiplash injury (chapter 6). During the examination, which involves the history, however, the mechanism of cervical pain must include this differentiation. Because the examiner must reproduce a painful sensation consistent with or similar to —if not exactly reproductive of—the initial complaint, this differentiation constitutes an important part of the examination.

Upon testing range of motion, active or passive, the evoked sensation must be ascertained by questioning the patient. The exact sensation must be described by the person when the examination is in process.

There is voluminous literature on the terms used by patients to describe their pain. Terms such as *excruciating, killing, devastating, overwhelming,* and so forth will, unless the accident is a major one, indicate an emotional reaction. Terms describing usual soft tissue pain are *aching, soreness, tension, boring,* and so forth and are elicited during the examination. Pain that is complained of without any examination, motion, position, or touch must be noted but again reconfirmed upon eliciting passive or active movement.

Nerve pain is usually of an electric sensation—sharp and often in a distal direction away from the neck. Head pain and face pain may alert the examiner to upper cervical segment neurologic involvement. Pain, numbness, tingling, or aching in the interscapular and upper extremity distribution implicates a possible neurogenic component.

The examination must carefully differentiate movement (active and passive) of the occipital cervical movement as compared with cervical motion. This is true in flexion-extension motion as well as rotation and lateral flexion. Where and when during the examination pain is felt *from* this motion is informative.

Tenderness also must be tested. Tenderness elicited over the upper cervical vertebral segment or at the base of the skull implicates cervical segment articular involvement in the former or neurogenic involvement in the latter.

In testing the lower segment (C-3 to C-7), lateral flexion must be remembered as never a *pure* motion but always with a component of rotation. Lateral motion followed by extension causes an approachment of the facets on that side with a concomitant closure (or opening) of the intervertebral foramina. Pain felt locally in this extension rotation movement implicates the facets, whereas when pain is felt in the upper extremity, it indicates possible nerve root involvement.

Limited flexion, with or without local pain, suggests ligamentous and extensor erector spinae muscle fascial tissue reaction. There may also be local tissue tenderness from pressure. Referred pain in the upper extremity from this forward flexion suggests nerve root traction or compression.

Extension of the neck and head causes compression of the posterior elements of the cervical functional units: compression of the articular facets, compression of the posterior annular fibers, and intervertebral foraminal closure. Local pain so elicited implicates soft tissue injury, whereas referred pain suggests nerve involvement.

It is apparent that in a meaningful examination the tissue involved is revealed or at least suggested by the descriptive terms used by the patient and by the maneuver that has elicited or aggravated the symptom, suggesting the mechanism by which the injury occurred and which tissue in the cervical spine is now mechanically involved. That the reaction is local and of soft tissue is proposed. That the reaction is neurogenic is also suggested. Other tests are explored in other sections of this text.

TRAUMA FROM TENSION

Tension means something different to patients, physicians, physiologists, therapists, physiatrists, psychologists, and psychiatrists. Regardless of the etiology of tension, the physical neuromuscular manifestation is similar. Tension within the neuromuscular system manifests a sustained *isometric* muscular contraction.

Isometric versus isotonic muscular contraction has been discussed in a previous section of this text.

> Muscular contraction specifically involves shortening of the contractile elements of the muscles but because muscles have elastic and viscous elements in series with the contractile mechanism it is possible for contraction to occur without an appreciable decrease in the length of the whole muscle. Such a contraction is called "isometric" (same measure or length). A contraction against a constant load with approximation of the ends of the muscle, hence shortening, is "isotonic." (Ganong)

Isometric implies that the muscle fibers contract with no shortening and thus no articular changes in the body; no motion occurs, but there is tension developed in the extrafusal fibers of the muscle. The tension from shortening generates all the chemical, electrical, and metabolic components of muscle contraction with all its component vascular aspects.

Muscular contraction is essentially a somatic-nerve-controlled activity in which the anterior horn cell of the spinal cord gray matter is electrically and chemically stimulated. Normally these contractions are under voluntary control to accomplish movement. A defective central nervous system such as a cerebral, midbrain, or cord lesion can cause uncontrolled muscular contractions known as spasticity. However, this latter muscular manifestation is not our concern here.

There is an intrinsic nerve control of muscular contraction that insures automatic coordination. When there is increased muscular contraction via alpha fibers of the somatic fibers from the anterior horn cells (Fig. 5–1), there is an acute contraction of the extrafusal fibers of the muscle group. The extent (force) of the contraction depends upon the number of motor fibers firing.

This coordinating factor which decides the number of muscle fibers contracting and the force generated must be appropriate with the intended task of that muscle group. The opposing muscles (antagonists) must relax appropriately. The reflex action of contraction and opposing muscle relaxation is termed

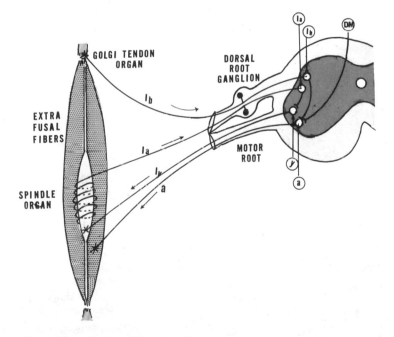

Figure 5–1. Pathways of spindle and Golgi systems to the cord. The spindle system supplies sensation to the cord via Ia fibers; the Golgi organs via Ib fibers. They end in the gray matter at cells Ia and Ib. The motor fibers to the spindle system are via I gamma fibers. These impulses "reset" the spindle system. The extrafusal fibers are innervated from the anterior horn cells (a) via alpha (a) fibers. Within the cord gray matter are numerous intercommunicating fibers. The upper cortical motor control is shown as DM.

reciprocal agonist-antagonist relaxation. The nerve pathways of this reciprocal relaxation have been well documented in neurophysiologic literature.

There must be a sensor mechanism that feeds the sensation back to the co-ordinating center to inform that center of the appropriate length and force generated by the coordinated contraction. This length and force must properly implement the intended action.

These sensor feedback pathways are mediated by the spindle cells in the muscle fibers and by the Golgi organs in the muscle tendon sites (Fig. 5–2).

In the *resting* muscle fibers (Fig. 5–3) there is no response of the Golgi organs transmitted to the cord via the Ib fibers since the tendon is not under tension.

Because the spindle system, even in the resting muscle, is under a slight degree of tension, there are impulses generated and directed to the cord via the Ia fibers. In the resting muscle there is a mild sustained tone in the extrafusal fibers but no discharge of alpha fibers.

When a muscle is stretched, actively or passively, the Golgi organs are stimulated and emit impulses to the cord via the Ib fibers. The spindle system is passively stretched and emits impulses to the cord. When the muscle contracts from an impulse directed to the extrafusal fibers via the alpha fibers, the Golgi organs are stimulated but the spindle system remains silent. In summary, activation of the Golgi organ system with transmission within the Ib fibers inhibits discharge of the spindle system via the Ia fibers from *control* center within the cord. This Golgi-spindle relationship insures the appropriate muscular contraction: either elongation or tension contraction.

Any muscular contraction must thus be appropriate for the intended task. There must be neither excessive nor inadequate contraction of the extrafusal fibers. The intrafusal fibers (spindle system) record the length as well as the rate of elongation. The Golgi organs record the tension (force). All are processed in

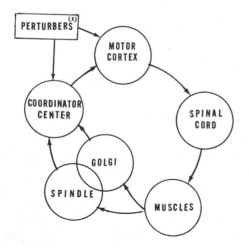

Figure 5–2. Nervous control circuit of the muscular system. The motor cortex initiates muscular action via the somatic system (spinal cord). The Golgi organs and the spindle system act as sensors that coordinate muscular action regarding length and force for appropriate action. *Perturbers* are extraneous factors (such as fatigue, anxiety, fear, anger, and so forth) that upset the fine coordination.

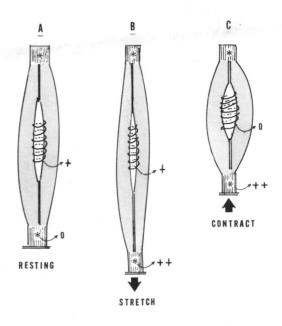

Figure 5–3. Spindle system coordination of muscular length, rate of contraction, and tension. (*A*) depicts resting muscle which, by its intrinsic elongation, activates the spindle system. (*B*) shows activity engendered in the Golgi organ by passive stretch with no spindle activity. In the actively contracted muscle (*C*), the spindle is relaxed and the Golgi strongly activated. The spindle and Golgi coordinate muscular action.

the coordinating system of the neurologic system at the cord level and are influenced by higher impulses from the cortex (Fig. 5–4).

Extraneous impulses influence the cycle. These are labeled *perturbers*. They can be beneficial in that they enhance the function of the system when an obstacle occurs. However, they usually are disturbances that disrupt or impair coordination of neuromuscular function. These perturbers include fatigue, peripheral mechanical stresses, pain, anger, emotional duress, anxiety, or depression. Their intervention upsets the proper balance of the neuromuscular coordinating system.

After contraction, muscles must relax. This means that the duration of the contraction, as well its intensity and force, must diminish or cease. This relaxation allows the restoration of internal blood flow, decrease of production of metabolites, and restoration of nutrients. If there is no period of relaxation, normal metabolism is interrupted.

The muscular increase in tone from emotional factors is not well-documented in the neurophysiologic literature. A postulated nervous system relationship is given in Figure 5–5.

That the emotions have influence from the hypothalamic-limbic system and that the limbic system has autonomic central nervous system manifestations is well-documented. These emotional messages are mediated to the hormonal and neuromuscular systems. It is the latter system that manifests to physiologic and ultimately the pathologic sequelae that is of interest here.

The autonomic nervous system reaction to limbic-hypothalamic stimula-

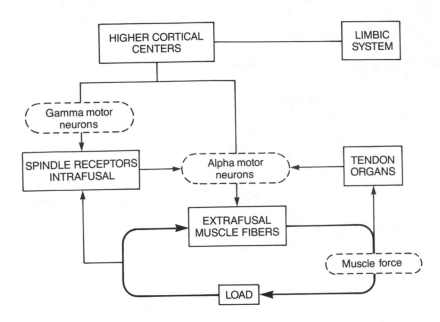

Figure 5–4. If there is an increase in alpha activity from the higher cortical centers (either voluntary effort or emotional stress), the extrafusal muscle fibers shorten and mechanically "unload" the spindle system. This disrupts the coordinated contraction of the alpha and gamma motor neurons. Both the alpha and the gamma motor neurons are activated by the higher centers and should be in harmony. The load is either actual or anticipated; in either case it influences the number of activated alpha motor neurons to the extrafusal muscle fibers.

tion from emotional trauma is primarily vascular with contraction (or relaxation) of *smooth* muscle throughout the body. These smooth muscles are found in the gastrointestinal, cardiovascular, and pulmonary systems. Contraction and relaxation of the blood vessels determine the degree of blood flow to all—including skeletal—muscles. Whether there is skeletal muscle contraction directly attributable to an autonomic nervous system motor impulse is conjectural (Denslow, et al), but there is skeletal muscle reaction to vascular tone and blood flow. There is also emotional control of the skeletal muscular system in the flight-or-fight manifestations of fear, anxiety, and anger.

The normal agonist-antagonist contraction and reciprocal relaxation of the somatic system is well-documented. The gamma loop nervous system also induces relaxation of antagonistic muscles. It may be the impairment of this gamma loop motoneuronal pool from limbic stimulation that causes the sustained isometric muscle tone of tension via the autonomic nervous system that results (Schmidt).

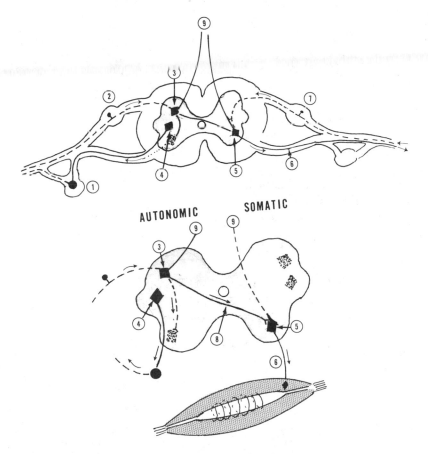

AUTONOMIC   SOMATIC

Figure 5–5. Autonomic-somatic cord level interaction. The fibers of the autonomic and the somatic nervous systems are shown: (*1*) the stellate ganglion, (*2*) the dorsal root ganglion, (*3*) sensory fiber nuclei within the gray matter, (*4*) motor cells of the autonomic system, (*5*) anterior horn (somatic motor) cells, (*6*) motor fibers to muscles, (*7*) somatic sensory fibers, (*8*) internal neuronal connections of the somatic autonomic systems, and (*9*) the cortical upper motor sensory neuronal connections. [The connection (*8*) remains unproven.]

When this emotionally induced isometric muscular contraction involves the neck muscles, all the manifestations of sustained isometric muscular contraction occur.

It must also be understood that sustained isometric contracture of the neck muscles can result from sustained postural positions as well as from nervous tension and that these postural positions may have a direct relationship to the emotions of the person. All aspects must be considered, but the end result is *sus-*

tained isometric muscular contraction of the cervical musculature.

Pain and tenderness can occur within the belly of a muscle as a result of an acute contraction or as a residual of a sustained muscular contraction, either isometric or isotonic. The isometric sustained contraction is more apt to cause ischemic pain because there is not the interim cycle of relaxation between contractions that permits evacuation of the residue metabolic substances and influx of new well-oxygenated blood.

Sustained muscular contraction in the neck, as in other parts of the musculoskeletal system, has been termed *tension myositis syndrome* (TMS) (Sarno). This has been considered to be a residue of emotional tension as well as of a sustained postural occupational syndrome causing muscular ischemia (Anrep, Barcroft).

Severe muscular exercise is known to cause muscular pain that may persist for several hours after cessation of the exercise (deVries). A *fatigue curve* has been demonstrated experimentally by a sensitive electromyographic instrument that has shown a decrease in the amplitude of the maximum voluntary contraction and an inability of the muscle fibers to relax (deVries).

The inability to relax is attributed to the disruption of the spindle system by the sustained contraction, elongation, and the ischemic changes. It is well accepted in sports medicine for musculoskeletal injuries that sustained stretching of the affected muscle for a period of several minutes results in a diminution or even cessation of pain. This is attributed to the reflex mechanism, in which the stretch of the tendinous Golgi apparatus (see Fig. 3–5) has been found to inhibit muscular contraction. The amplitude of electromyographic muscular contractions diminishes when the involved muscles are stretched (Norris, et al). The Golgi reflex *unloads* the spindle system of the muscle. Once unloaded and relaxed, the muscle no longer produces metabolic by-products of contraction, the mechanical ischemia (sustained contraction) is diminished, greater venous flow occurs, and there is an increase of oxygenated blood to the muscle.

The metabolites secreted by contracting muscles that remain to become local irritants as well as nociceptors are "factor P," potassium shift, and lactic acid.

It is a well-accepted clinical experience that local heat, massage, ultrasound (deep heat), and stretch decrease muscular tension pain (TMS), which explains the ischemic concept. Medications causing relaxation also decrease muscular tension pain, and most relaxant medications are psychic tranquilizers rather than pure muscle fiber relaxants. This indirectly confirms that emotional tension causes sustained muscular tension, which in turn causes pain from ischemia and accumulation of metabolites (Fig. 5–6).

Strong isometric contractions have been shown to invoke muscle fiber tears with microscopic tearing and some formation of edema. The inflammation of the periosteum, by which muscles attach to bone, and its subperiosteal tissues also results in pain and local tenderness.

Sustained muscular contraction also causes sustained intervertebral disk

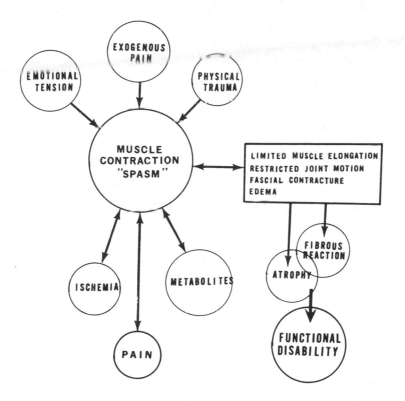

Figure 5–6. Cycle of pain causing spasm with evolution to functional disability.

compression. This sustained disk compression, just as sustained compression of cartilage, diminishes the ability of the mucopolysaccharides to imbibe nutrient fluid and thus ultimately to cause disk degeneration. There are numerous causative factors that cause disk degeneration, which will be discussed in a subsequent chapter, but unrelenting sustained compression upon the disk without release is probably a significant factor.

As in any cartilage tissue—which the intervertebral disk is—normal nutrition requires intermittent relaxation after compression. Expansion of the cartilaginous tissue mechanically imibes the nutrient solutions from the joint-space tissue fluid. Sustained prolonged compression of the disk will inevitably compress the tissue fluids *out of solution,* and failure to relax and so to allow expansion will inhibit imbibition. The collagen and the mucopolysaccharide matrix thus undergoes degeneration, and loses the hydraulic effect of the disk, as well.

Degeneration and dehydration of the intervertebral disk also allows the pedicles and the zygapophyseal joints to approximate. The foramen narrows.

These mechanical changes are the result of disk degeneration and are the ultimate mechanical effect of external muscular compressive forces.

Internal disk pressure has been shown to cause diskogenic pain either from pressure upon the outer annular fibers or from pressure upon the posterior longitudinal ligament. Sustained isometric muscular contraction of the cervical spine muscles compresses the disk and causes protrusion of the nucleus, with subsequent bulging of the annulus. This can result in pain. A magnetic resonance image (MRI) would reveal this condition.

Used for the purpose of initiating muscular relaxation to come under voluntary control, biofeedback has been effective treatment to relieve tension myositis. Inasmuch as biofeedback demonstrates a diminution of involuntary motor units on the electromyographic tracing with resultant decrease in pain, it strongly suggests that the pain was caused by sustained muscular contraction.

Another aspect of biofeedback uses skin thermal changes from vasomotor hypertonicity. Learning to control vasomotor reaction with resultant decrease in musculoskeletal pain also suggests that vasoconstriction is a cause of muscular pain and that sustained muscular contraction may be a component of vasomotor ischemia (Birk, Taylor).

The diagnosis of tension as the cause of the musculoskeletal symptom of pain is made from the patient's history and a careful examination. The person reveals the relationship of pain ensuing from an emotionally tense situation, for example, personal professional situation. The diagnosis of tension as the cause of musculoskeletal pain must never be one of exclusion; that is, asserting that tension is responsible when no other cause can be found. The statement "it's all in your mind because you are tense" is an accusation, not a diagnosis.

"I get tense from pressure at work," "When I get upset, my neck gets tense and I get a stiff neck and a headache," "My husband is so demanding that I get upset and my neck begins to hurt," "I get in 'knots' when we argue," "When I get angry, my neck 'acts up,' " "My neck gets sore and stiff from pressures at work, and my chiropractor tells me my neck is 'stiff' and out of line," "I cannot turn my head without pain after an argument with my son," "My job is very demanding and I get stiff necks that really hurt"—these are all typical statements in a history of a patient suffering from cervical pain from emotional tension. The relationship of neck symptoms from an emotionally induced tense situation can be elicited. The patient will frequently also associate the symptoms with emotional stress. This association aids in making the diagnosis and assists in ultimately orienting the patient for a constructive beneficial therapy program.

The examination begins with the appearance of the individual. Tension is depicted in the attitude; the mannerisms; the manner of speech; the postural attitude of anger, tension, anxiety, or depression. The patient's use of certain words in the history alerts the examiner to the presence of anxiety or tension. The patient's descriptive words can convey a great deal of meaning. The sensation of muscular pain can be described as *tense, tight, in knots, lumps, deep aching,* or *burning.*

The examination is now both of actively and passively examining the neck and often of reproducing the pain. A standard aspect of a musculoskeletal examination is determining the *range of motion* (ROM). ROM is not synonymous with normal motion. Range of motion of the neck is the degree of motion elucidated by passively moving the neck and observing at what level of the cervical spine and at which direction of motion there is limitation. The controversy in determining the reason for loss of ROM is whether the limitation is from structural changes in the joints, changes in the soft tissues, or from protective muscle spasm incurred as a sequela of pain, anxiety, or fear.

There are no fixed, firm criteria establishing which of these factors is the cause of limited ROM. Often a careful passive testing of ROM determines whether there is *protective* limitation imposed by the patient from fear, reaction to pain, or anxiety. In this case the limitation of ROM gives the examiner a certain feel of restriction. Some *give* can be achieved during the examination through distraction or by performing the test with the patient in various positions.

The restriction of motion in any specific direction or motion is informative. If the limitation is in *all directions of motion* and throughout the entire range, a question is raised as to which tissues can possibly restrict *all* motion. Limitation in all directions throughout the entire range is unanatomic, inasmuch as it involves all tissues—ligaments, joint capsules, and all muscles in the cervical spine. Such limitation implies that it is muscle *guarding* that limits motion and restricts normal range. The most common such muscular limitation is tension caused by anxiety, fear, apprehension, or concern about pain.

In the examination the normal ROM of the upper cervical segment (occiput-atlas-axis) as well as of the lower cervical segment (C-3 to C-7) must always be kept in mind. Both passive and active motions must comply with the expected normal motion for each segment.

When there is total limitation and unyielding of restriction to any degree throughout all levels of the cervical spine, the examiner must conclude that the limited range is guarding from pain, anxiety, fear, and apprehension. This guarding may be unintentional reflex action and should not imply malingering but, rather, merely limited range of motion not caused by structural ranges in the cervical spine. It is the responsibility of the examiner to ascertain the reason for the patient's guarding.

The history of how long the restriction has been noted by the patient is important. A brief, recent, limitation after a trauma is understandable, but persistent limitation after no ascertainable injury is indicative of guarding from tension.

Restricted ROM at the end points of joint motion implicates restriction imposed by joint capsular tightness as well as limitation of muscle fascial elongation. This limitation imparts a springy feel to the examiner: a brief rebound reaction to attempted motion. The reaction has a doughy feeling upon passive motion, and the restriction from active ROM confirms the probable etiology of emotional tension.

Reaching the end point of ROM may be *uncomfortable* but, gently done, not particularly *painful, excruciating, killing, terrible, horrible,* or *unbearable.* In an apprehensive individual who is guarding the ROM as a result of anxiety or fear, such pain or discomfort is claimed throughout all movement, at all points of the range, and in all directions, and may elicit all the above descriptive terms of pain sensation.

Passive range of motion limitation from *a slipped disk* or a *subluxed verte-bra* without commensurate trauma or x-ray evidence is untenable and should not be so stated to an apprehensive patient.

X-ray examination that reveals a straightening of the cervical lordosis indicates muscle *spasm,* which must be differentiated from the position of the patient during the x-ray examination and should be clinically confirmed. Frequently there is a tendency to *overread* x-ray findings; that is, to assume that x-ray findings are evidence of pathology rather than confirmation of the clinical suspicion. It must never be forgotten that x-ray examinations provide confirmatory revelation or confirmation of the suspected clinical findings and that x-ray findings, per se, may be misleading.

Diagnosis of cervical tension myositis must be a true diagnosis, never an accusation or a casual deduction because no organic pathology can be found.

Tension, either emotional or postural, can be considered a trauma to the cervical spine and can cause pain and impairment. The factors revealed from the history and the examination suggest neuromuscular skeletal dysfunction. Our discussion thus far has focused on emotional tension as the trauma. Now we can concentrate on tension myositis from posture.

Limited range of motion due to cervical *arthritis* does not fall under the category of limitation from tension; it will be discussed in chapter 8 dealing with degenerative arthritis.

TRAUMA FROM POSTURE

The concept of trauma in the cervical spine from posture alteration may elude the average practitioner. Faulty posture does impart trauma to numerous aspects of the musculoskeletal system, especially to the vertebral column. Trauma to the cervical spine from faulty posture is a frequent cause of pain and disability.

To review posture briefly as related to the cervical spine, *normal cervical posture* can be defined as the cervical lordosis assumed and maintained in holding the head directly within the center of gravity.

Normal posture implies:

1. there is essentially minimal or no muscular activity needed to support the head

2. the intervertebral disks maintained in proper alignment experience no excessive anterior or posterior vertebral disk annular compression
3. the nucleus remains in its proper physiologic center
4. the zygapophyseal joints are properly aligned and do not bear excessive weight upon the body assuming the erect posture
5. the intervertebral foramina remain appropriately open and the nerve roots emerge with adequate space.

Improper posture affects all of these factors and impairs effortless balance, with resultant pain and impairment. Posture must be evaluated in the standing, sitting, and functioning body. In proper posture maintaining the head in the center of gravity, the head is held by ligamentous, fascial, disk pressure, and joint capsule support. Only isometric muscle tone supplements these supporting tissues.

The proper erect posture has been discussed in chapter 1. The head is only slightly anterior to the center of gravity with the meatus of the ear as a superior point on the line of gravity. This center passes through the curve of the cervical lordosis and descends anterior to the atlanto-axial joints and through the lowest cervical vertebrae.

Because the head is held slightly anterior to the center of gravity the tissues that prevent forward downward rotation must be the posterior musculature and the posterior ligamentous structures. These tissues act in a static manner, with the ligamentum nuchae playing a major role. The erector spinae musculature acts in an isotonic effort to diminish the stress upon the ligaments.

Proper Standing Posture. Over the years there have been numerous texts devoted to the topic of proper standing posture. Evolution has been documented, as have the basic neuromuscular mechanisms. Approximation to the center of gravity has been postulated to be the *ideal* posture with the minimum of curvature away from the center. In essence, to maintain proper physiologic posture the head must be maintained effortlessly at the apex of the cervical spine at the center of gravity with a minimum of cervical lordosis.

Not only must this axiom apply to the cervical spine, but also it must apply to the thoracic and lumbar curvatures. There must be a minimum of dorsal kyphosis and lumbar lordosis. An excess of either of these two curves makes its impression on the superincumbant curve of the cervical spine (Fig. 5–7).

A *forward head posture* incurred from an increased dorsal spinal kyphosis places the head ahead of the center of gravity. The head of an average adult weighs in the vicinity of 8 to 12 pounds. If the head is considered to weigh 10 pounds and is held 3 inches ahead of the center of gravity, the head now essentially "weighs" 30 pounds (Fig. 5–8). Because there is an increase in the cervical lordosis, each functional unit also increases its lordotic angle. This increase approximates and compresses the posterior aspect of the disk (Fig. 5–9).

Besides neck strain with all its sequelae, there are other bodily changes that cause impairment and discomfort (Fig. 5–10). The shoulders *droop* in that the scapulae rotate downward, the breasts sag, the thoracic cavity is diminished with resultant decreased vital capacity, and the person is literally shorter in height.

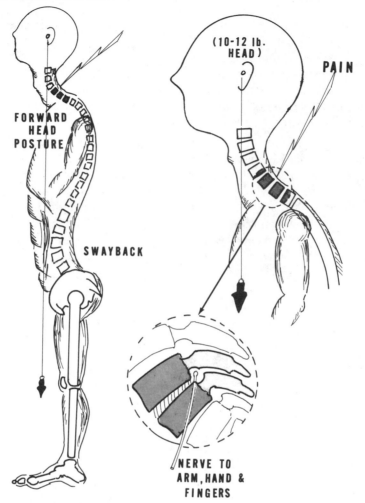

Figure 5–7. Forward-head posture rejuvenation strategy. When the head is held ahead of the center of gravity (forward-head posture), the 10-to-12-pound head causes an increase in lordosis and a closing of the posterior foramina, thus entrapping the nerve roots.

Of these sequelae, the drooping shoulder posture adversely influences the cervical spine. The upper trapezius muscle originates from the cervical spine and thus the depressed scapulae place muscular strain upon the neck. The forward-head posture also initiates symptoms of the shoulder-upper extremity-thoracic outlet syndrome that poses a differential diagnostic consideration in evaluating the exact cause of upper extremity neurologic radicular symptoms.

Assuming a forward-head posture by bending forward at the waist and bringing the head to a horizontal vision position physiologically increases the

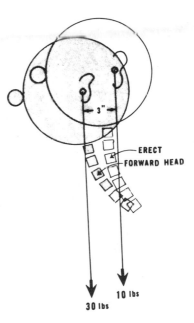

Figure 5–8. Weight of the head in forward-head posture.

cervical lordosis. This assumed position, per se, decreases the normal active and passive rotational ROM. A person can normally decrease the ability to turn the head to the right or to the left by assuming an exaggerated forward head posture. In that intentionally assumed forward head posture there is a loss of 25 to 50 percent normal rotation to each side. This is a physiologic loss of ROM without any discomfort.

This posture, however, can become pathologic when it is maintained persistently. In this pose the zygapophyseal (facet) joints become maximally weight bearing and their cartilage is exposed to persistent recurrent trauma.

In this increased cervical lordotic posture the intervertebral foramina are closed and the nerve roots are potentially compressed.

With prolonged unremitting compression from the posture, the zygapophyseal joint capsules can become constricted and even adherent, thus leading to gradual structural limitation. With cartilaginous structural changes, a degenerative arthritic condition of the facet joints occurs. If there is also superimposed muscular tension, the compression is increased and structural tissue changes are precipitated.

There are many activities of daily living (ADL) that incur this posture and must be recognized and corrected before irreparable changes occur. To name only a few, the use of bifocal glasses, faulty sitting posture—especially in front of a computer (Fig. 5–11)—prolonged standing posture required in many occupations (Fig. 5–12), so that daily flexibility exercises must be recommended (Fig. 5–13).

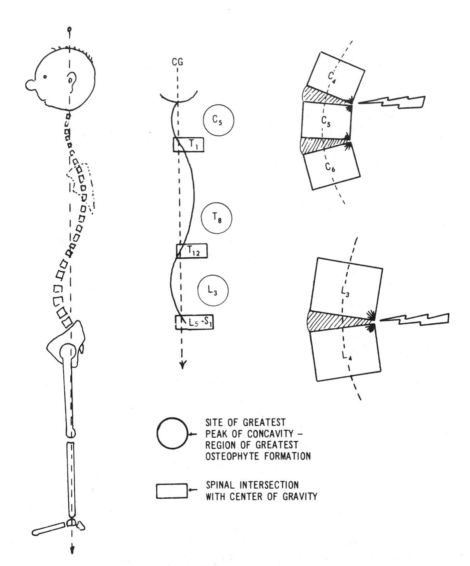

SITE OF GREATEST
PEAK OF CONCAVITY –
REGION OF GREATEST
OSTEOPHYTE FORMATION

SPINAL INTERSECTION
WITH CENTER OF GRAVITY

Figure 5–9. Sites of greatest osteophyte formation. The lateral view of the static erect spine (posture) demonstrates the sites of transection of the spine with the plumb line of gravity (external ear meatus, odontoid process, T-11, T-12, and sacral promontory). The greatest points of pressure, thus the sites of osteophyte formation, are at the points of greatest concavity, farthest from the plumb line (C-3, T-8, L-3).

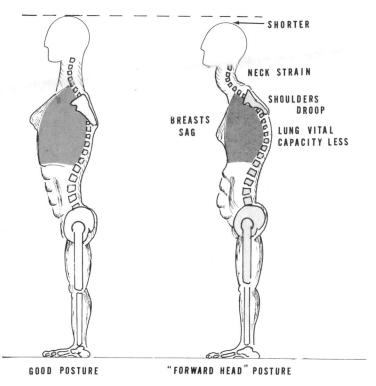

SHORTER

NECK STRAIN

SHOULDERS
DROOP

BREASTS
SAG

LUNG VITAL
CAPACITY LESS

GOOD POSTURE   "FORWARD HEAD" POSTURE

Figure 5–10. Painful sequelae of forward-head posture rejuvenation strategy. In addition to the effects upon the cervical spine, the female breasts sag, the shoulders droop, there is a shortening of erect stature, and there is a decrease in vital lung capacity.

It is interesting that the condition of temporomandibular joint arthralgia (TMJ syndrome) is now considered to be related to and aggravated by the forward head posture as well as by deep-seated emotional tension. These factors—tension and faulty posture—contribute to the dental malalignments and constitute the current concept that must be incorporated into proper treatment of TMJ syndrome.

The posture of depression is essentially that depicted in the forward-head posture. The dejected attitude and the depressed muscular activity of this psychiatric condition incur all the pathologic aspects of the forward-head posture and, by causing pain and physical impairment, aggravate the condition of emotional depression. Merely treating depression with psychotherapeutic drugs and psychotherapy are not sufficient. All the aspects of faulty and thus pathologic pain- and disability-producing posture must also be addressed and remedied.

Therefore, accepting trauma as a causative pain-producing cervical prob-

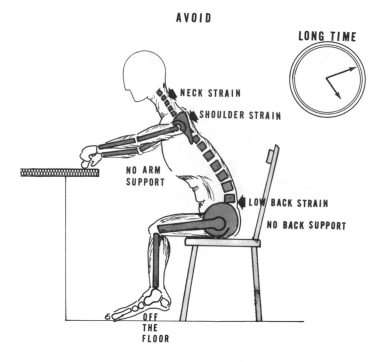

Figure 5–11. Faulty sitting posture creates cervical stress.

lem, the traumata of faulty posture combine with the trauma of tension. Postural tension implies that the extensor muscles of the cervical spine must be in sustained isometric contraction to support the head in its ahead-of-the-center-of-gravity position.

Because of this posture, the normal supporting structures (the internal disk pressure, the intervertebral ligaments, the ligamentum nuchae, and so forth) now must be supplemented by sustained isometric muscular contraction of the extensor musculature. This muscular action is a compensatory muscular activity that is initiated by the neurologic mechanisms discussed earlier. The extrafusal muscular fiber contraction is gravity initiated and sustained and the normal physiologic neuromuscular reaction gradually becomes pathologic.

The third trauma has been stated to be *subluxation* from external forces: the so-called *whiplash* injury will be discussed in the next chapter.

AVOID

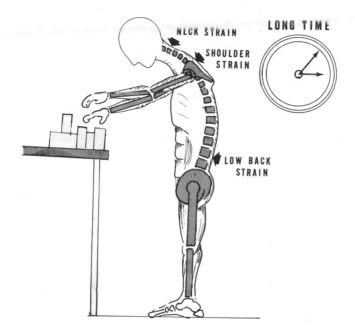

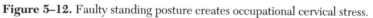

Figure 5–12. Faulty standing posture creates occupational cervical stress.

AVOID

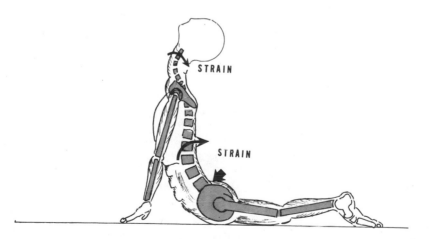

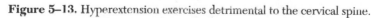

Figure 5–13. Hyperextension exercises detrimental to the cervical spine.

BIBLIOGRAPHY

Anrep, GJ and Saalfeld, EV: The blood flow-through skeletal muscle in relation to its contraction. J Physiol 85:375, 1935.

Barcroft, H and Millen, JLE: The blood flow-through muscle during contraction. J Physiol 107:518, 1948.

Birk, L: Biofeedback: Behavioral Medicine. Grune & Stratton, New York, 1973.

Campbell, HJ: Correlative Physiology of the Nervous System. Academic Press, London, 1969.

Denslow, JS, Korr, IM, and Krems, AD: Quantitative studies of chronic facilitation in human motoneuron pools. Am J Physiol 150:229, 1947.

deVries, HA: Physiology of Exercise, ed. 3. William C. Brown Pubs, Dubuque, IA, 1980.

Farfan, HF: The scientific basis of manipulative procedures. Clin Rheum Dis 6(1):159, 1980.

Ganong, WF: Review of Medical Physiology, ed 7. Lange Medical Publications, Los Altos, CA, 1973.

Henry, JP and Stephens, PM: Stress, Health and the Social Environment: A Sociobiological Approach to Medicine. Springer-Verlag, New York, 1977.

McMahon, TA: Muscles, Reflexes and Locomotion. Princeton University Press, Princeton, NJ, 1984.

Norris, FH, et al: An electromyographic study of induced and spontaneous muscle cramps. Electroencephalogr Clin Neurophysiol 9:139, 1957.

Sarno, J: Mind over Back Pain, William Morrow and Co., New York, 1984.

Schmidt, RF (ed): Fundamentals of Neurophysiology, ed 2. Springer-Verlag, Berlin, 1978.

Taylor, LP: Electromyographic Biofeedback Therapy. Biofeedback and Advanced Therapy Institute, Los Angeles, CA, 1981.

CHAPTER 6

Subluxations of the Cervical Spine: The Whiplash Syndromes

Hyperflexion and hyperextension injuries of the cervical spine are termed universally *whiplash* injuries. However, the term remains controversial, enjoying no universal understanding or acceptance of its definition.

Whiplash injuries have become commonplace in the medical and legal arenas. Its victims enter the courts, where the plaintiffs and their lawyers attempt to receive adequate compensation for the resultant pains and disabilities. Insurance carriers are inundated with these claims and assert that the numerous compensations for these injuries are the cause of increasing exorbitant insurance rates.

This condition occurs increasingly in western societies where the automobile is the predominant means of transportation. The condition is noted more in metropolitan regions and is a major cause of lost employment time. The incidence is higher in women than in men (5 to 1) and in the age group of 30 to 50 (Su and Su).

The symptoms from these injuries last more than 6 months in 75 percent of the patients who lose an average of 8 weeks of work.

The term *whiplash,* applied to hyperextension injuries, was coined by Dr. Harold Crowe in 1928. In the original description, the effects of sudden acceleration-deceleration upon the neck and upper body from a forceful external impact were described as resulting in a violent "lashlike effect." The term *whiplash* was used essentially to describe the effect of external trauma. The tissue damage causing the symptoms resulting from mechanical impact has gradually become what is meant by the medical diagnostic term—whiplash.

Controversy remains, however, with regard to its analysis. Saternus postulated that "this diagnosis should take into account anatomic and mechanical aspects" and should be limited to "violent *dislocating* force of acceleration (deceleration) of the stationary axial skeleton causing 'typical' effects on the unrestrained head and neck" with resultant "severe stretching of the soft tissues, the intervertebral joints, nerve roots, and peripheral nerves in the posterior cervical regions of the spine" (Fig. 6–1).

In essence, Saternus's definition describes a joint *luxation* or *subluxation* causing a strain-sprain injury upon the periarticular soft tissues (Fig. 6–2).

Whiplash is considered to be an injury of soft tissue from acceleration-deceleration, essentially a *strain-sprain* type of injury. Contrary to *whiplash, strain-sprain* has been defined and generally accepted.

The term *strain* is defined in *Stedman's Medical Dictionary* as injury resulting from overuse. *Sprain,* from the Latin *exprimere* (to press out) is defined as an injury to a joint with possible rupture of some of the ligaments and tendons without dislocation or fracture. From the Latin *dis* (apart) and *locatio* (a placing), *dislocation* is described as "a disarrangement of the normal relation of the bones entering into the formation of a joint." This is otherwise termed *luxation.*

There is a paradox here because it is difficult to visualize a "sprain" causing rupture to a ligament of a joint that has not exceeded its normal range of mo-

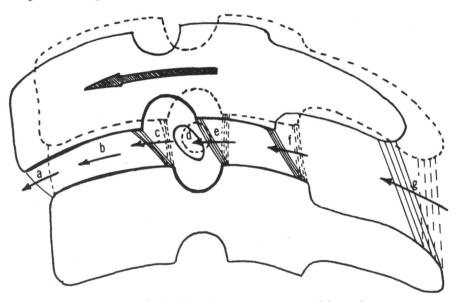

Figure 6–1. Tissues involved in hyperflexion sprain injury of the neck.

a   =   anterior longitudinal ligament
b   =   intervertebral disk
c   =   posterior longitudinal ligament
d   =   nerve root
e   =   ligamentum flavum
f   =   interspinous ligaments
g   =   nuchal muscles

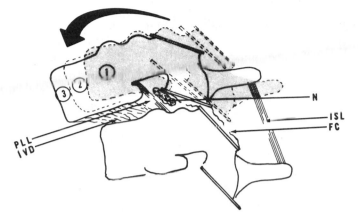

Figure 6–2. Hyperextension-hyperflexion injury. Normal physiologic flexion (1 to 2) is possible with no soft tissue damage. When motion is exceeded (3), the intervertebral disk (IVD) is pathologically deformed, the posterior longitudinal ligament (PLL) is strained or torn, the nerve (N) is acutely entrapped, the facet capsule (FC) is torn or stretched, and the interspinous ligament (ISL) is damaged.

tion— a "luxation" or a "subluxation." By their very definitions luxations and subluxations are derangements of the opposing joint surfaces. If a whiplash is a severe sprain, it must be assumed that there has been a luxation or a subluxation.

It is a prevalent thought that the whiplash syndrome is essentially or predominantly an acceleration injury with a secondary deceleration injury. A rebound phenomenon is postulated, with flexion following extension (or vice versa when the original injury is from flexion). Hyperextension need not follow hyperflexion, nor must hyperflexion follow hyperextension. Either or both may occur and need to be documented by a careful history.

Crowe claimed that "dynamic injuries of the spine cause a genuine pathological insult that causes prolonged distress and disability, often lasting for several years after the accident." Bosworth is more sanguine, stating, "The neck is not a whip. . . . This diagnosis is vague and thoroughly unscientific. . . . There is a tendency for this terminology to be employed . . . through lack of sufficient knowledge to make a specific diagnosis. . . . The term to the honest is merely a bulwark behind which ignorance skulks; to the dishonest [it is] a mirage with which to confuse and deluge." Munro stated, "In its pure form and when rightly diagnosed, the symptoms of 'whiplash' injury are those of cervical muscular spasm often complicated by neurosis."

Forces of deceleration or acceleration may be linear translation, lateral translation, rotational, compressive, or a combination of these forces. Numerous ergonomic studies have provided scientific data regarding the forces experienced (Severy; Mertz and Patrick; McGhee). By accurate history the effecting force must be documented to determine the tissue(s) affected.

The symptoms allegedly resulting from this type of injury are vaguely described, but all can be attributed to nociception from injured soft tissues; in this case, the cervical spine. Johkees claimed, "Victims have recovered very well from all the other fractures and lesions the accident caused and have gone back to normal work and life with them, but . . . it is often the 'symptomless' drama of the strained neck that needs the appropriate treatment [for recovery] of the soft tissues of the neck."

The tissue sites of nociception in the cervical spine have been discussed in Chapter 2, but a brief review for pertinent reaction to external stress is appropriate at this juncture.

The tissues of the cervical spine that contain innervation capable of transmitting pain have been summarized:

1. Anterior longitudinal ligament
2. Outer layers of intervertebral disk annulus
3. Posterior longitudinal ligament
4. Nerve root dura
5. Capsule of the zygapophyseal (facet) joints
6. Intervertebral ligaments
7. Extensor musculature
8. Posterior longitudinal ligament
9. Flexor musculature: the colli and scalenes

The precervical fascia may also be a nociceptive site, especially where it is traversed by the sympathetic nerves. All these tissues will receive appropriate discussion later in this chapter.

The external neck muscles are implicated. Selecki divided neck injuries into several categories. Injuries he termed *mild* resulted in hyperextension injury to the longus colli and the scalene muscles. *Moderate* injuries sustained tears of the longus colli and scalene muscles as well as of the anterior longitudinal ligament. In this severity of injury the esophagus, larynx, intervertebral disks, the nerve roots, and even the vertebral arteries and their intrinsic innervation may exhibit trauma with resultant symptomatology. In the category of *severe* Selecki included tearing of the disk annulus, nerve root damage, and possible contusion of the brain stem.

The most commonly expressed complaints after a whiplash injury are:

1. Neckache—pain of various description and intensity
2. Neck "stiffness" with limited movement
3. Headache
4. Shoulder pain—often of interscapular site
4. Neck tenderness
5. A complaint of "spasm."

There may be subjective and objective evidence of nerve root radiculopathy. The complaint of nerve root irritation—dermatomal or myotomal radiation—implies possibly more significant injury. All these symptoms will receive individual consideration and evaluation as an indication for therapeutic intervention.

Because the condition, and thus the symptoms, have been considered to be psychogenic by many and to be a pathologic tissue injury by others, a discrepancy remains to be clarified. Hohl and Lipow attempted this differentiation in several reports.

EVALUATION OF THE MECHANICAL INSULT TO THE CERVICAL SPINE

It has been aptly stated that the direction and intensity of the force and the conditions of the person during the accident have a significant impact upon the expected pathologic residual. "The mechanism of injury is of major importance in the complete understanding of spine trauma." (White and Panjabi)

The position of the person's head is instrumental when reconstructing the accident. Was the person facing straight ahead or turned to one side? This implies the direction of the movement that the head and neck translated.

A direct forward head position implies that the head moved in a vertical direction, that is, in flexion or extension or both. The intensity may also be ascertained by the ultimate disposition of a person's head gear, eye glasses, and so forth.

With the person's head turned to one side, a lateral and rotatory torque force and ultimate spine movement can be reconstructed. No pure lateral movement of the spine is possible without a simultaneous rotational movement. The tissues involved in this forced movement are different from those in a pure vertical flexion-extension motion.

The expectation of the person receiving the impact must be ascertained insofar as he or she is prepared and thus is contracting protective muscles to absorb the intensity of the impact. The alertness and awareness of the person at the time of the accident thus is a significant part of the history.

The direction, and to a certain degree the intensity, of the impact can be ascertained by a careful history and often can be confirmed by radiologic studies (Harris and colleagues). There are numerous laboratory studies that simulate cervical injuries of the type sustained by the patient, and the correlation is gradually adding credence to the complaints of the injured person.

The spine has been analyzed by numerous medical specialists as being of two columns (White and Panjabi; Holdsworth; Louis), but others see it as three columns and having vector forces in movement. The column concept indicates the tissues of the cervical spine that move with various movements, normally and pathologically, of the head and neck. This has been discussed in chapter 1 as well.

The two-column concept defines the anterior column as comprising the (1) vertebral bodies, (2) the intervertebral disk, (3) the anterior longitudinal ligament, and (4) the posterior longitudinal ligament. These are the anterior verte-bral supporting structures of the spine.

The anterior longitudinal ligament, amply innervated to be a site of nociception, is inelastic but may avulse from its bony attachment to the ver-tebrae. As the anterior longitudinal ligament circumscribes a large part of the anterior and anterlateral aspect of the vertebra, it comes close to the emerging nerve roots. If it becomes injured and swollen, the adjacent nerves may be affected.

Ahead of the anterior column, and yet not essentially considered to be a part of the column, are the anterior (flexor) muscles. They flex the spine and are injured when the neck hyperextends. These neck flexor muscles are divided into three layers:

1. Superficial: the sternocleidomastoid and trapezius muscles
2. Intermediate: splenius capitis, levator scapulae, longissimus capitis, semispinalis capitis, iliocostalis cervicis, scalenei, and the rhomboid
3. Deep: rectus capitis, superior and inferior oblique capitis, prevertebral longus capitis, and longus colli

Any or all of these muscle groups can sustain injury from an extension in-jury, depending on the force of the insult.

The posterior column consists of

1. The posterior osseous structures of the neural arch (the laminae, pedi-cles, transverse processes)
2. The zygapophyseal joints
3. The ligaments: posterior longitudinal and interspinous
4. The erector spinae muscles

Within the posterior column are contained the nerve roots and their dural containers.

The ligamentum nuchae and ligamentum flavum are elastic and thus may stretch, avoiding significant injury to elongating forces when the posterior col-umn is distracted. The interspinous and supraspinatus ligaments are relatively inelastic and thus may tear when excessively stretched.

Pure flexion-extension indicates movement in the coronal plane. In these motions the components of the anterior column are compressed and those of the posterior column distracted. Hyperextension causes the exact opposite, that is, the anterior column distracts and the posterior column compresses. Several ways of expressing this concept are used: *compressive hyperextension, compressive hyperflexion, distraction hyperflexion,* and *extension without compression or distraction.* These can be considered physiologic kinetic terms with clinical significance.

A *three-pillar column* concept has been expounded (Louis) in which the anterior column is the same in the two-column concept, but the posterior column contains the bilateral laminae and (zygapophyseal) facet joints. The three-column concept applies more directly to the lower cervical segment

(C-3 to C-7). This three-column concept may be more understandable and acceptable because within the posterior column are located the foramina that open and close asymmetrically in lateral and rotational motion (see Chap. 1).

In understanding the mechanisms of cervical injuries the following motions pertain:

1. Flexion
2. Extension
3. Hyperflexion
4. Hyperextension
5. Flexion-rotation
6. Extension-rotation
7. Lateral flexion
8. Vertical compression

Each of the above types of motion has a precise resultant injury that is discernible from history and examination, and frequently may be confirmed from radiologic studies.

Because there are emerging nerve roots from the foramina of the lower cervical segments, a radicular history, confirmed by examination, and resultant radiculopathy may occur. The upper cervical segments do not lend to this Injury Mechanism Classification, and each of the upper units has limited motion, direction, and differing nerve root emergence and distribution (see Chap. 1).

THE WHIPLASH INJURY: HISTORY AND PHYSICAL EXAMINATION

The whiplash injury can be classified according to the acute phase or the chronic phase. It can also be clinically classified as mild, moderate, or severe.

In a rear-end collision the trunk of the patient reacts immediately to the rear-end impact and deforms in the forward movement. The car decelerates as does the patient's trunk, but the head extends upon the cervical spine at the upper segment. This passive motion occurs at the occipital cervical junction and the upper cervical units C-1 to C-2. Almost instantaneously the lower cervical segment C-3 to C-7, T-1 extends (Fig. 6–3).

The forces expended in this impact have been computed by numerous experimental models. If the speed of the rear car is between 9 and 15 miles per hour, a force of 5 Gs can be generated.

The forward movement of the shoulders and the subsequent head-neck extension occur within 400 to 500 milliseconds, and the initial neck motion occurs within the first 250 milliseconds, that is, a quarter of a second.

The neck flexors involved in a mild impact probably are the superficial muscles: the longus colli and the scalenes. The anterior longitudinal ligament

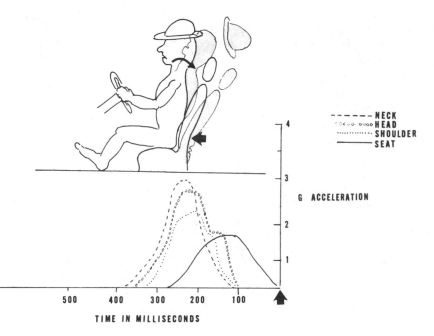

Figure 6–3. Upper body-neck deformation in rear-end collision. With a force from behind, the head, neck, and shoulders deform at different points in time—all happens in less than 0.5 sec.

may also be extended. The muscles undergo abrupt elongation with possible microscopic tearing resulting in microscopic intrinsic hemorrhage and edema (Braaf and Rosner).

The muscle spindles are also abruptly elongated, and the reflex relationship of the intrinsic and extrinsic muscle fibers becomes disassociated (Fig. 6–4).

The immediate symptom may be discomfort in the anterior portion of the neck. A headache may occur, which may be due to the initial abrupt motion of the occipital-axis and the atlas-axis articulation, with irritation of the branches of the greater occipital nerves (Bogduk, 1980). Precervical edema may cause a slight dysphagia and even some minor speech impediment.

The abrupt neurologic reflex from the intrinsic nerve supply—the spindle system—may account for the difficulty many patients claim in being unable to lift their heads from the pillow the next morning and from the neck weakness elicited in the examination.

The delay in symptoms frequently reported by the patient is probably related to the gradual effusion and microscopic hemorrhage in the neck flexor muscles. Failure to resolve this effusion and microscopic hemorrhage during the early acute phase may account for the evolution into chronic stages with

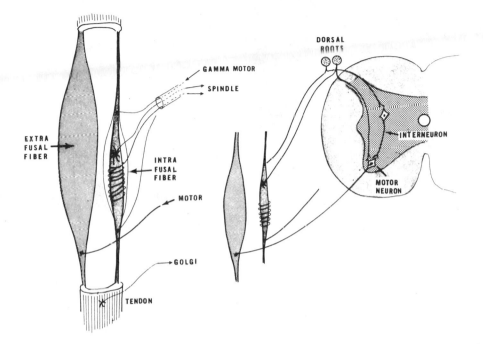

Figure 6–4. Muscle spindles. The contractile fibers are known as extrafusal fibers and are innervated by the motor neuron. The intrafusal fibers contain the spindles which end in annulospiral fibers and flower-spray endings. These fibers send impulses to the cord, conveying stretch responses. In voluntary extrafusal contraction there is no stretch reflex. In an abrupt contraction of the extrafusal fibers, such as a tendon jerk, there is a reflex via the interneuron that stimulates the motor neuron. The tendon stretch is mediated through the Golgi tendon organ. The gamma motor fibers adjust the length and thus the response of the spindle system.

persistence of limited range of motion.

The anterior longitudinal ligament also may be elongated and may be responsible for the referred interscapular pain so frequently claimed by the injured patient (Cloward). The cervical nerve roots that pass the anterior longitudinal ligament laterally and through the scalenes are probably responsible for many of the vague radicular symptoms such as numbness and tingling of the hands and fingers.

The sympathetic branches of the anterior primary divisions of the nerve root emerge through the precervical fascia. Stretching and subsequent edema in that vicinity explain the sympathetic symptoms claimed by the patient, including blurred vision, dysphagia, vertigo, and light-headedness (Fig. 6–5).

The inflamed edematous muscles account for the restricted neck motions. This limitation is also explained by the impaired spindle system reflexes. Diffi-

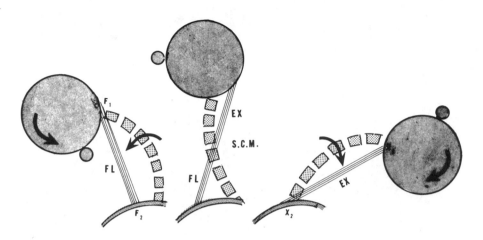

Figure 6–5. Muscular reaction to *whiplash* injury. *(Center)* Sternocleidomastoid (SCM) muscle in extension (EX) to upper half of cervical spine and flexor (FL) to lower half. *(Right)* Hyperextension, the SCM is completely an extension and shorter than in neutral. *(Left)* In flexion, the SCM is completely flexor and shorter than neutral and hyperextension. This rapid movement overstretches muscle and causes a reflex inhibition and muscle strain.

culty in swallowing may occur due to precervical edema. This edema may be noted in careful study of soft tissue shadows of routine lateral cervical spine x-rays.

The inflamed edematous muscles undergo irritation contraction, that is, *spasm*. This spasm, an acute reflex contraction of damaged muscle fibers, further enhances the intrinsic pathology.

If the injury is moderate to severe, other deep tissues may become involved. For example, the anterior longitudinal ligament may be avulsed from the vertebrae, and the annular fibers of the intervertebral disk may undergo tearing (Fig. 6–6).

In the acute, mild case of whiplash (80 to 90 percent of most reported cases) the signs are minimal or absent except for finding "trigger areas" of tenderness in the superficial muscles and the measurable limited range of neck motion. Most symptoms are subjective. X-ray films may reveal "straightening of the cervical lordosis," the significance of which is unacceptably objective to most clinicians.

In moderate to severe cases there are both subjective and objective neurologic signs indicating nerve root involvement. Here the neurologic signs indicate which root, which dermatome, and which myotome are involved. Labora-

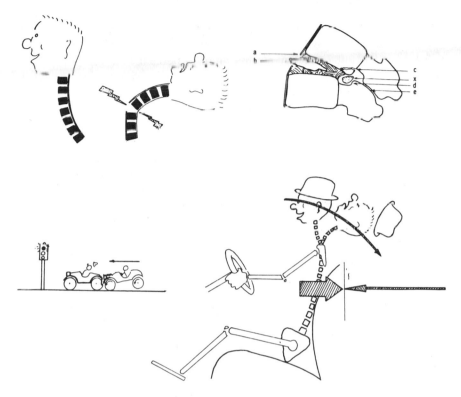

Figure 6–6. Rear-end impact with neck hyperextension sprain. When the patient is at a standstill, the impact from the rear causes an acute hyperextension movement of the neck. Possible injuries are (a) anterior longitudinal tear, (b) anterior herniation of intervertebral disk, (c) chip fracture of vertebral body, (d) facet encroachment into foramen, and (e) acute facet impingement. The nerve root, x, can be impinged by this movement.

tory tests such as magnetic resonance imaging (MRI), computerized tomography (CT) scans, and electromyography (EMG) are confirmatory.

There are clear guidelines about when and under which circumstances radiographs should be considered after an acute cervical injury. When there is evidence of significant neurologic deficit, there is no question that an x-ray examination is indicated. But in mere *posttraumatic neck pain* without subjective or objective radicular signs—that is, when the injury is considered essentially soft tissue strain-sprain—x-ray examinations are usually not considered to be beneficial.

In a recent review of 351 patients seen in an emergency room situation and prospectively studied regarding the outcome of posttraumatic neck pain, workers (MacNamara and associates) concluded that in only 2 percent of the x-ray examinations was there revealed proven fractures or significant ligamentus injuries. In their conclusion, they revealed that 52 percent of the patients ultimately underwent radiologic studies, and 66 percent had litigation, both of which apparently incurred radiologic studies. Their conclusion suggested that litigation required x-ray studies but also revealed a small percentage of positive findings in otherwise negative examinations.

Inasmuch as some injuries occur in older people, there may be evidence of pre-existing structural changes in the cervical spine such as disk degeneration, neural (foraminal) spurring, and some degree of spinal stenosis. A careful history should confirm whether previous injuries existed or neurologic changes, that makes this an aggravation of a pre-existing condition.

The diagnosis, made carefully and thoroughly and explained succinctly and understandably to the patient, is the beginning of appropriate treatment.

Acute Mild Injury

The patient must be told what has happened and what is causing the symptoms, what the treatment will be and what is expected from the treatment. The patient must be expected to participate actively in the treatment, and he or she must be given the reason for participation.

Because this medical condition has been widely discussed in the newspapers, on television, in the parlor, around the neighborhood, and by "experts" alike, and because it has a reputation for being severe, difficult to treat, persistent if not incurable, and because, unfortunately, it requires so much documentation for possible legal compensation, clear discussion and explanation to the patient are *mandatory*. This is the first and possibly the most truly important aspect of treatment.

Treatment must be initiated early—preferably within hours, no longer than a few days. Treatment must be aggressive but gentle. It must be remembered that the injury has caused soft tissue injury with inflammation, edema, and possibly microscopic hemorrhage. A severely sprained knee, ankle, or shoulder receives this consideration; why not the sprained neck?

The medical literature is replete with "standard" treatment protocols. Heat rather than ice; ice rather than heat; rest rather than activities; early exercise rather than rest; traction; ultrasound; manipulation; transcutaneous electric nerve stimulation (TENS); collar; local injections; acupuncture; and medication to diminish inflammation, to allay anxiety, to decrease muscle spasm, to relieve pain, to prevent disuse, to prevent contracture, and so forth. Each has its advocates, proponents, and critics.

A careful evaluation and understanding of the tissue changes that have occurred must be the basis for proper treatment. The acute phase is that of a severe sprain. Resultant edema and possible microscopic hemorrhage must be thought to have occurred. Nociceptive chemicals—histaminelike, prosta-

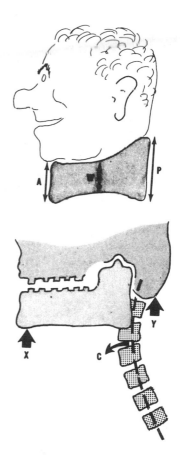

Figure 6–7. Soft cervical collar. Made of felt or similar material, the collar is narrower in the front and supports the chin so that the patient leans upon it, thus keeping the head in a slightly flexed posture. The posterior portion is wider and acts merely as a reminder, by contact, to prevent extension. This collar functions by kinesthetic touch rather than by physical restraint or support.

glandins, substance P, and kinins—accumulate at the injured site.

Immediate *rest of the part is indicated*. A well-fitted felt collar (Fig. 6–7, 6–8) may support the head upon the neck and *splint* the parts. This must be prescribed as an adjunct to other therapy. As acute inflammation is apparent, ice administered early decreases pain, decreases blood vessel dilatation, intervenes upon the formation of histaminelike by-products, and thus diminishes further formation of edema and hemorrhage.

Prolonged use of ice becomes painful, as it causes vasoconstriction and additional local ischemia. Within a day the use of heat, rather than ice, is physiologic to remove the accumulated nociceptors gradually.

Heat also prevents the unwanted binding of the intersecting collagen fibrils of the capsules that lead to contracture. Heat causes vasodilation and increases blood supply to wash out the accumulating toxins. Heat is also sedative and soothing.

Prolonged use of a collar is contraindicated (Cammack). Within several

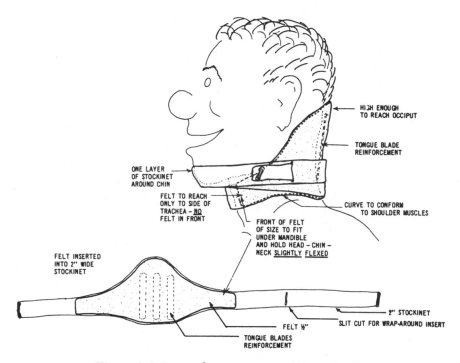

Figure 6–8. Pattern for construction of felt neck collar.

days (3 to 4) the collar becomes addictive; dependency develops. Immobilization allows the organization of the inflamed tissues to indurate muscles, fascial planes, and periarticular tissues (Mealy and associates).

Active and carefully guided passive range of motion is indicated. Active and possibly forceful manipulation is, unfortunately, often applied in the early stage. When there has been no subluxation, with overriding and locking of the facet joints, manipulation can only cause further tissue injury or insult and thus should be avoided.

Gentle mobilization (rather than manipulation) is indicated early. Here mobilization or even gentle manipulation is best administered according to the concepts of Maigne that indicate movement in the direction *away* from pain or restriction rather than manipulation in the limited or painful direction (Fig. 6–9). The difference between manipulation and mobilization is a subtle point. Long lever *end point thrust* is to be condemned. Short lever thrust (Maitland) is also not indicated but, rather, gentle mobilization, that is, passive assisted range of motion is indicated. It must be remembered that the goal of treatment is to *regain pain-free movement*.

The value of traction still remains unproven. Traction of the degree that

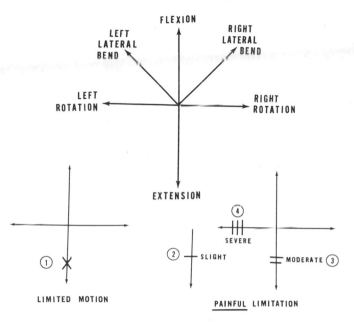

Figure 6–9. Recording of range of motion of cervical spine. X indicates mere limitation and no pain (1) and lines are placed for restriction and simultaneous pain (2 to 4).

supports the head on the neck and gently decreases the lordosis (10 to 15 lbs) and separates the facets of joints may be of value. Usually traction cannot be applied for sufficient time to accomplish this purpose. Alone it is valuable when the injury has been severe or when there has been subluxation, but for the mild acute whiplash most traction is not tolerated, accepted, or beneficial.

When the acute phase has subsided but muscle spasm and joint limitation persist, the failure of acute treatment is apparent. Traction now may be necessary to overcome periarticular contracture.

Subacute Phase: Mild. The subacute phase can be considered to begin when the acute initial symptoms begin to wane. This is usually a matter of several days in a relatively mild injury. There remains tenderness and limitation of motion. Some degree of active movement now is possible, albeit slightly uncomfortable and unpleasant. It must be explained to the patient that this discomfort is to be tolerated as a process of restoration of the range of motion. Passive motion in the mild subacute phase is greater than in the acute phase.

Active motion is indicated now. This implies that active exercises are to be initiated. Exercises are to be of small gradual increments of amplitude done four times a day. Ice applications should precede the exercises, and heat should follow. Ten to fifteen minutes of ice and the same duration of heat usually suffices. Both can be applied in the form of Hydrocollator pads (cold and hot).

The purpose of exercise is to increase flexion, extension, rotation, and lateral flexion actively. Exercises done *by* the patient cannot be harmful inasmuch as the therapist *is* the *patient*, who will only "go so far" (Figs. 6–10, 6–11). The *translation exercise* (Fig. 6–12) not only increases the range of motion but also institutes the sensation (feel) of the proper posture, which aids in the teaching of proper posture in ADL.

The exercises to gain range of motion must be followed by exercises to increase the strength of the muscles (Figs. 6–13, 6–14).

The strengthening exercises are done isometrically. *Isometric* indicates contraction and *holding* of that contraction of the neck muscles with *no* active range of motion. The muscles contract and relax, thus *massaging* all the accumulated toxic substances of inflammation without causing potentially painful joint motion. Muscle fibers are also strengthened.

A too frequently neglected aspect of treating a neck injury and preventing the possibility of recurrence or persistence of symptoms is the failure to improve the posture of the individual (Figs. 6–15, 6–16).

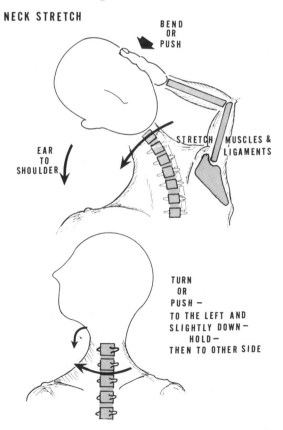

Figure 6–10. Neck stretch exercise.

SITUP: STAGE 1

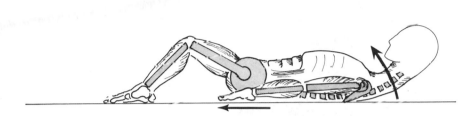

Figure 6–11. Neck flexor strengthening during partial sit-up

A forward-head, rounded upper back posture causes increased lordosis and excessive weight bearing on the neck. The posterior zygapophyseal joints are compacted, the posterior annular fibers of the disk are compressed, and the foramina are narrowed. All these encroach upon the nociceptive tissues, causing pain and impairment.

Correcting posture requires conscious effort by the patient with exercises, but only modification of the person's concept of good posture and daily effort toward achieving it will result in good posture as an unconscious habit.

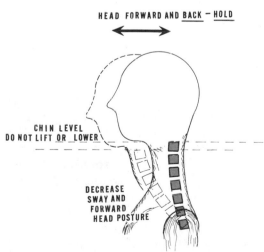

Figure 6–12. Translation exercise.

NECK STRENGTHENING 1

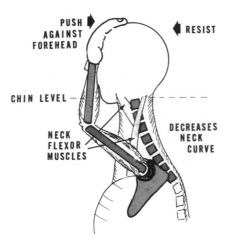

Figure 6–13. Neck strengthening exercise (1).

Activities of daily living must be evaluated and modified to avoid any position that can aggravate the patient's cervical condition or prevent healing after an acute injury. These are numerous and should be addressed by a competent occupational therapist, who can evaluate the patient's specific daily activities. One frequent daily activity that is often performed improperly is sitting in a chair. Proper sitting posture is shown in Figure 6–17.

There are many other exercises (Figs. 6–18 to 6–23) that influence the range of neck motion and correct posture. These are to improve trunk and shoulder flexibility and strength as well as to teach the feel of proper posture throughout the entire body. These can be included in the daily-exercise period or, preferably, done during the recommended frequent daily one-minute breaks.

This one-minute break indicates pulling away from one's task for a brief period and doing the exercise. These exercises require no change of attire, no loss of time from work, no perspiration, and, in addition to improving flexibility of the anatomic part being stretched, allow relaxation of the person from the intensity of his or her task.

Medication indicated during the acute phase of mild cervical injury needs to be addressed. It must be stressed that unnecessary medication is to be avoided. Certain medication can cause dependency or even addiction.

Pain may be severe but not usually. Anxiety is prevalent and tends to intensify the severity of the pain or to increase the implications of the severity of the injury. Anger from the accident—Why did this happen to me? My new car is damaged—may intensify the patient's perception of discomfort.

NECK STRENGTHENING 2

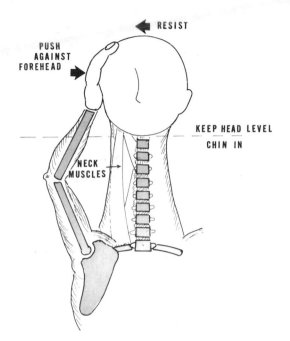

Figure 6–14. Neck strengthening exercises (2).

Litigation, unfortunately, also intensifies the symptoms. A well-meaning attorney wishes to dramatize the severity of the accident to ensure maximum compensation. To this is often added the delay of payment by the insurance carrier or the insensitivity of the primary attending physician. Anger intensifies the muscular tension, aggravates the postural component, and adds to the depression, which decreases the voluntary efforts of the injured person.

Medications often are prescribed to relieve pain, to decrease muscular tension, or to decrease inflammation. All are of value if given in a limited, judicious manner over a limited duration with careful periodic reviews to determine whether they are still effective or even needed. An explanation of the role of drugs and their potential side effects is mandatory to assure patient cooperation and compliance.

A proper evaluation of the tissue injury dictates which medication to prescribe. Knowledge of the person's emotional state and reaction to the injury influences the medication and its dosage. An explanation of the cause and extent

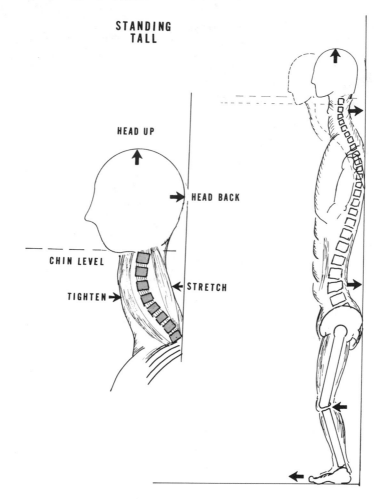

Figure 6–15. Standing tall.

of the injury frequently decreases the need for medication or at least the strength and the duration of its prescription.

Acute Severe Hyperextension Injury

A *severe* hyperextension injury implies significant tissue injury far exceeding that of the mild acute injury.

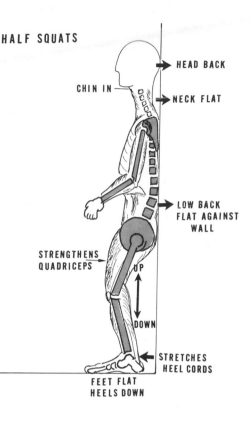

Figure 6–16. Posture exercise: half squats.

In this injury there may be:

(1) Tear or avulsion of the anterior longitudinal ligament

(2) Tear of the anterior flexor muscles

(3) Tear of the annular layers of the intervertebral disk. This latter injury, the tear of the annular fibers of the disk, is discussed in Chapter 7.

Hyperextension injury may include:

1. Hyperextension dislocation
2. Avulsion fracture of the anterior arch of the atlas
3. Extension teardrop fracture of the atlas
4. Fracture of the posterior arch of the atlas
5. Laminar fracture
6. Traumatic spondylolisthesis
7. Fracture-dislocation (Harris and colleagues).

Any of these is diagnosed with appropriate x-ray studies, and each requires specific medical, orthopedic, or neurosurgic attention. *To suspect is to study.* To study is to diagnose and thus to ensure proper treatment. The possibility of any

IDEAL SITTING

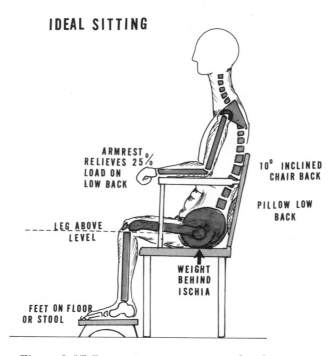

ARMREST RELIEVES 25% LOAD ON LOW BACK

10° INCLINED CHAIR BACK

PILLOW LOW BACK

LEG ABOVE LEVEL

WEIGHT BEHIND ISCHIA

FEET ON FLOOR OR STOOL

Figure 6–17. Proper sitting posture to avoid neck strain.

SHOULDER STRETCH

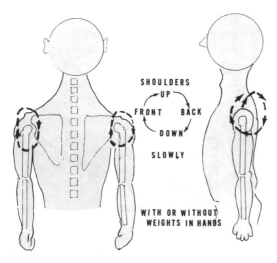

SHOULDERS
UP
FRONT   BACK
DOWN
SLOWLY

WITH OR WITHOUT WEIGHTS IN HANDS

Figure 6–18. Shoulder stretch.

THE ONE MINUTE BREAK:
STANDING PUSHUP

HANDS
HIGHER
THEN
LOWER

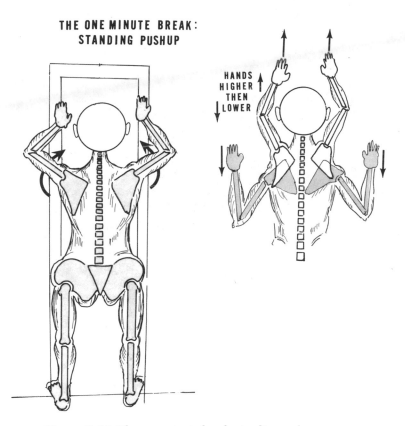

Figure 6–19. The one-minute break: standing push-up.

of these injuries is the indication for performing routine x-ray examinations of an injury even though the severity, at first, is undetermined.

Hyperflexion Injuries

An injury to a person incurred by a vehicular force from the front results in reflex action, causing acute flexion of the cervical spine and consequential different tissue injuries, symptoms, and findings (Figs. 6–24, 6–25).

The classification of acute cervical spine injuries (Harris and associates) can be itemized as follows:

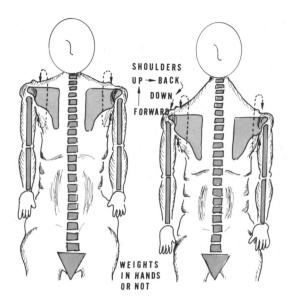

Figure 6–20. Shoulder blade range of motion.

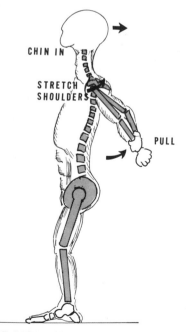

THE ONE MINUTE BREAK: SHOULDER STETCH 1

Figure 6–21. The one-minute break: shoulder stretch 1.

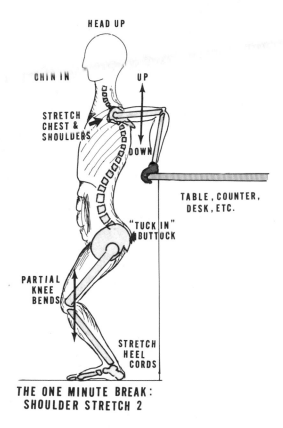

HEAD UP

CHIN IN

STRETCH
CHEST &
SHOULDERS

UP

DOWN

TABLE, COUNTER,
DESK, ETC.

"TUCK IN"
BUTTOCK

PARTIAL
KNEE
BENDS

STRETCH
HEEL
CORDS

THE ONE MINUTE BREAK:
SHOULDER STRETCH 2

Figure 6–22. The one-minute break: shoulder stretch 2.

1. Flexion
   a. Anterior subluxation
   b. Unilateral interfacetal dislocation (Fig. 6–26)
   c. Bilateral interfacetal dislocation
   d. Simple compression fracture
   e. Avulsion fracture of the spinous process (C-6, C-7, or T-1)
   f. Complete luxation with disruption of the posterior ligaments, the facet capsule, and the annular disk fibers. Some fragmentation of the vertebral body may occur.
2. Flexion rotation
   Injury can result in a further classification in which there is rotation as well as flexion. This mechanism may result in a unilateral facet dislocation (Fig. 6–27).
3. Vertical compression
   As in any trauma mechanism, there can be a component of compression as well as linear flexion or extension (Figs. 6–28, 6–29), and the sequelae

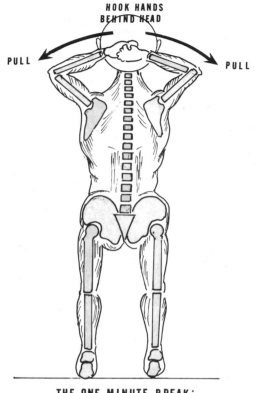

**THE ONE MINUTE BREAK:
SHOULDER STRETCH 3**

Figure 6–23. The one-minute break: shoulder stretch 3.

differ in that there can be noted

a. compression (burst) fracture of the atlas

b. compression fracture of any cervical vertebra (Fig. 6–30).

Most of these injuries are noted from appropriate x-ray studies. Further clarification is possible with planigrams or CT scans. The suspicion or confirmation of a fracture dislocation mandates a thorough neurologic examination and further studies such as MRI. A neurosurgic or orthopedic consultation is also warranted.

Mild Acute Flexion Injury. An acute flexion injury causes anterior compression of the anterior column (vertebrae and anterior disk annular structures) and distraction of the posterior column components.

The tissues that sustain injury are essentially those included the two columns. The interspinous and supraspinous ligaments are elongated. They are resilient, so tearing is rare in mild injuries, but some ligamentous injury undoubtedly occurs. It has been estimated that 50 percent undergo delayed insta-

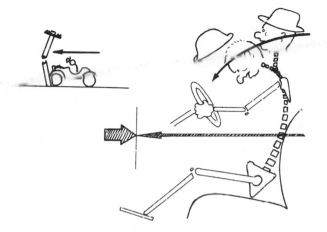

Figure 6–24. Flexion vehicular injury. Flexion phase of acceleration injury to the neck (sprain). The body stops suddenly, but the neck continues due to continued momentum. The neck flexes and in fact may hyperflex. Possible injuries are (a) an acute synovitis due to subluxation of the articular facets, (b) capsular tear of articulation, (c) posterior nuclear herniation, and (d) posterior longitudinal ligamentous tear. All these may cause injury to the nerve root. The flexion phase of injury may be isolated, may follow as a "rebound" of an extension injury, or may be followed by a hyperextension phase.

bility (Chesire).

The extensor muscles can be *overwhelmed*. This implies that they are hyperelongated before their spindle system reacts appropriately, allowing the extrafusal fibers and their fascial compartment to undergo trauma (Figs. 6–31, 6–32).

The facet joints undergo minor subluxation, and cause no frank dislocation, merely a capsular elongation.

The anterior annular fibers undergo compression and the posterior annular disk fibers, elongation. The posterior longitudinal ligament is also elongated.

The nociceptive-containing tissues are the erector spinae muscles, posterior ligament, posterior longitudinal ligament, facet capsules, and the outer annular fibers. Pain is felt locally in the neck and is referred in the distribution of the myotomes and dermatomes.

Many have stated that the "typical" whiplash injury has a reflex rebound component of flexion immediately following a hyperextension injury. The opposite is also claimed, that is, that hyperextension follows the hyperflexion injury. Both may occur, but the reflex reaction rebound is probably the lesser of the incidences and causes less tissue injury.

It must also be noted that many vehicles struck from behind, thus causing a hyperextension injury, are secondarily propelled into a vehicle ahead, resulting

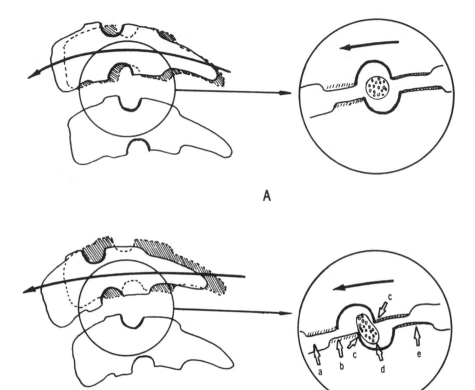

Figure 6–25. Mechanism of hyperflexion spray injury to the neck. *(A)* Normal forward gliding of the upper vertebra upon the lower and its effect upon the intervertebral foramen. *(B)* Hyperflexion with disk distortion, (a) foramen distortion, and nerve root impingement, (d) anteriorly-inferiorly by the lower uncovertebral joint and superiorly-posteriorly by the upper articular facet, (c) the articular facets are subluxed (e).

in a second flexion injury. The history substantiates this double injury to both anterior and posterior tissues.

Symptoms, Findings, and Treatment. Pain and tenderness is felt posteriorly in the erector spinae muscles and in the insertional area of the upper trapezius muscles. Neck flexion is painful and limited, as is rotation. Treatment is essentially the same as that of the acute hyperextension injury.

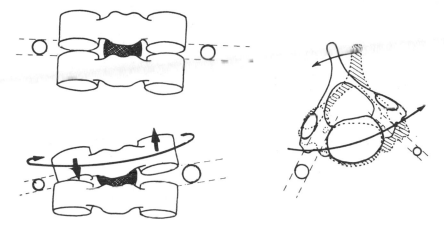

Figure 6–26. Unilateral subluxation from excessive rotation (unilateral facet impingement or dislocation).

Posttraumatic Headache

Headache following a whiplash injury is not infrequent. This is probably due to (1) insertion of trapezius muscle; and/or (2) subluxation of the occipital cervical segment.

Head and upper neck pain at the occipital and cervical insertion of the upper trapezius fibers will be further discussed in the section on myofascial pain. It is sufficient here to state that the upper trapezius muscle becomes tender and nodular (Fig. 6–33). The site of insertion, also the emergence site of the greater superior occipital nerve, becomes a tender zone (Figs. 6–34, 6–35).

The headache symptoms are also attributed by some authors (Bogduk, 1979) to subluxation of the occipital-atlas-axis articulation (the upper cervical segment) (Fig. 6–36).

Headache, better termed cephalalgia, is a discomfort in the forehead, scalp area, or the base of the skull. There are numerous causes of headache, but here we concern ourselves only with the cephalalgia of post whiplash, the occipital neuralgia.

Headaches can occur from irritation of the cervical extensor muscles as well as from reflex tension of the occipital muscles. *Trigger points,* areas of muscular nodularity, are found in the sternocleidomastoid, splenius capitis, temporalis, and masseter and trapezius muscles, which refer pain to the occipital area (Fig. 6–37).

Hunter and Mayfield claimed that the posterior ramus of C_3 was crushed between the posterior arch of the atlas and the lamina of the axis as a result of

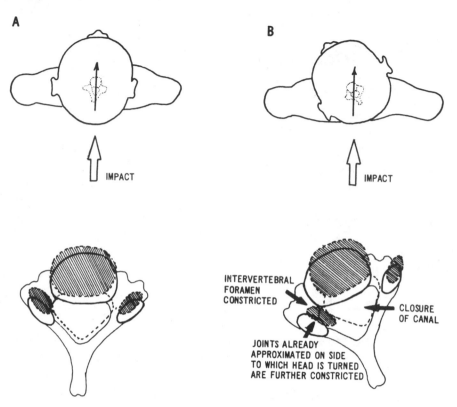

Figure 6–27. Effect of deceleration injury to neck with head turned. (A) The "to-and-fro" movement of flexion and extension of a deceleration injury with the head facing forward. (B) With the head rotated to the left, the forward glide causes constriction of the foramen on the side toward which the head is turned. The foramen is already smaller (physiologically) on that side, and the joints are already in closer proximity. The spinal canal also undergoes greater deformity; thus more strain upon the spinal cord may result.

excessive extension of the head. This was coupled with simultaneous rotation of the head.

Bogduk clearly demonstrated that the nerve cannot be anatomically compressed by this maneuver. The idea, commonly expounded, of compression of the greater occipital nerve at its exit point below the mastoid between the fibers of the upper trapezius and the sternocleidomastoid muscle was also refuted (Bogduk, 1980).

Bogduk postulated the following sequence of the mechanism of occipital neuralgia: The C_2 ganglion lies under the posterior arch of the atlas, medial to the articular capsule of the lateral bodies of the atlas and the axis. The nerve then branches into the dorsal and the ventral rami, which supply sensory fibers to the capsule of that joint.

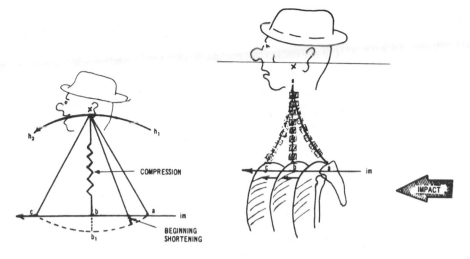

Figure 6–28. Compression theory of *whiplash* injury. The impact is taken by the body, which moves horizontally (im). The head does not move either up or down or forward or backward. The length of the neck at rest (before impact), x–a, shortens to length x–b at the moment when the head is vertically above the body. At this midpoint the length of the neck should be x–b_1; therefore, at this point there is compression. At the end of the impact movement, the neck regains its full length, x–c (equal to x–a). The diagram on the left shows the pathway of the neck when the mechanism is that of neck movement upon the body, h_1–h_2 (see Fig. 6–25). The length remains the same throughout the entire arc and at best causes traction upon the cervical spine.

The cervical injury of a whiplash violently subluxes that joint (atlas-axis), causing excessive capsular stretch. The dorsal root of the greater occipital nerve as it penetrates the joint capsule becomes inflamed and refers pain into the dermatomal region of that nerve root (see Fig. 6–35).

Treatment. Treatment is similar to that for hyperextension injuries, namely, ice, followed by heat, massage, mobilization, and medication. A trial of manual, then mechanical, traction can be begun, as well as acupuncture, TENS, and so forth. Local injections into the trigger zones have their advocates, as does the technique of "spray stretch" (Travell and Simons). Whereas epidural injections of steroid and anesthetic agents have been widely used in lumbar radiculopathy, there is a current reference to the successful use of this technique in cervical pain and radiculopathy (Warfield and others).

Posttraumatic Vertigo

There are many causes postulated for posttraumatic vertigo. After an acute hyperflexion-hyperextension cervical injury many patients complain of vertigo

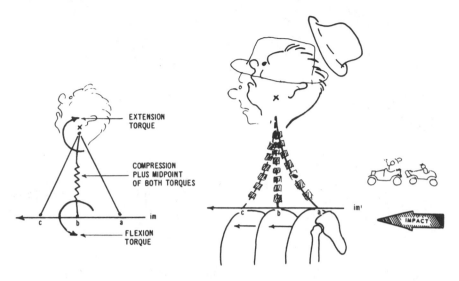

Figure 6–29. Compression-plus-torque theory of cervical injury resulting from *whiplash*. The impact is taken by the body, which moves forward horizontally (im). Similar to Figure 6–28, there is compression of the cervical spine when the head is directly over the body at the midpoint of the impact reaction. In contrast to Figure 6–28, the head is elevated and rotates *(torque)*. The extension torque of C and the flexion torque of C-7 place the avulsion stress in the midcervical region.

as well as headache, nausea, and occular discomfort. The specific diagnostic procedure to determine the cause remains unclear and the treatment remains difficult.

Unbalance of the sympathetic nervous system has been postulated for years as the cause. This imbalance is attributed as the cause termed *Barré-Liéou syndrome.* This sympathetic traumatic imbalance has in turn been attributed to trauma to the sympathetic fibers that accompany the vertebral arteries, and therein has been the claim that mild subluxation compresses the vertebral arteries in the atlas-axis region (C1-2). Excessive rotational forces exceeding physiologic rotation of the atlas-axis articulation has been postulated.

When there is a concomitant vertebral artery insufficiency from atherosclerosis or a congenital anomaly, vertigo is more common. The presence of osteophytes has also enhanced vertebral artery compression in the mid and lower cervical regions, because osteophytes are not usually present in the atlas-axis region.

A recent article (Tomita and colleagues) documented dynamic entrapment of the vertebral artery by the ventral branch of the second cervical nerve. This entrapment was confirmed by arteriography and alleviated by surgery.

When posttrauma vertigo persists and is significant *and* can be influenced

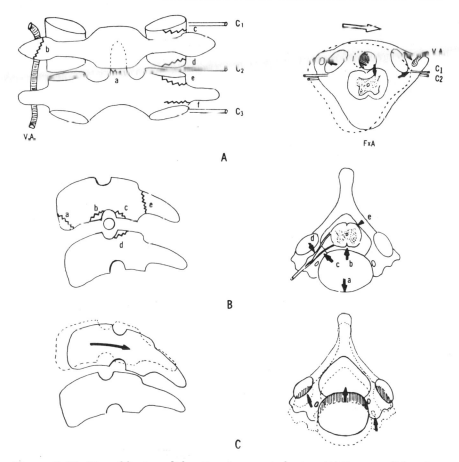

Figure 6–30. Sites of fracture-dislocations in e cervical spine. *(A)* Fracture-dislocation sites: a, odontoid process; b, process; c–f, articular facets of atlas-axis. *(B)* Fracture sites: letters show corresponding sites in both views. *(C)* Posterior dislocation sites (bilateral).

by active or passive manual rotation of the upper cervical segment, vascular studies are indicated. This possibility also signifies that manipulation in the presence of vertigo is contraindicated until adequate studies are performed.

Acute Central Spinal Cord Injury

In evaluating the neurologic sequelae of any hyperextension, hyperflexion, or excessive rotational deformation of the cervical spine, trauma to the cord must be considered as well as injury to peripheral nerve roots. The *acute central spinal cord injury* is a significant neurologic syndrome that may result.

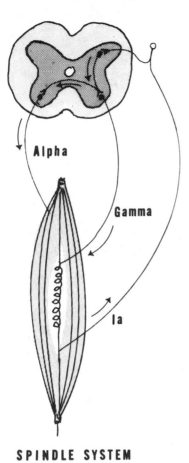

SPINDLE SYSTEM

Figure 6–31. The spindle system. The spindle system of the muscle moderates the tone of the extrafusal fibers. It transmits the information to the cord via Ia fibers at the cord level, where it modifies the tone of the extrafusal muscle fibers (innervated by somatic alpha fibers). The spindle system is "reset" to the appropriate tone via the gamma fibers.

Patients have been documented as sustaining severe neurologic deficit after a hyperextension-hyperflexion cervical injury with minimal or even insignificant alteration of vertebral alignment on radiologic studies. Any degree of luxation may have occurred, with return to proper vertebral alignment, but there may still be resultant cord compression or angulation.

Symptoms. The syndrome of acute central spinal cord injury reveals subjective and objective evidence of central nervous system dysfunction. The usual history is that the patient has not struck the head nor lost consciousness. He or she is fully aware of the incident in some detail, other than just that the head and neck were "snapped."

Immediately after the injury the patient feels numbness of the entire trunk and/or extremities and is able to move neither arms nor legs. There may be a tingling sensation, and coordination, if any extremity function exists, may be

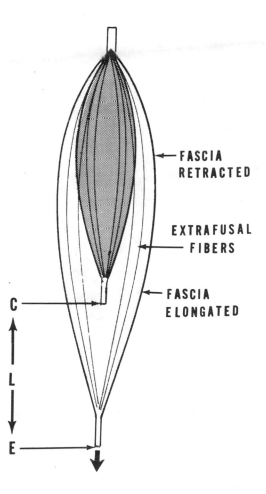

Figure 6–32. Fascial limits to muscular elongation. Any muscle bundle can elongate to the extent that its fascial sheath permits. The extrafusal fibers elongate fully, but the fascia must be passively elongated. Fascial contracture restricts muscular elongation and joint range of motion. L = length, C = contracted, E = elongated.

impaired.

Findings on Examination. Neurologic examination reveals hyperactive deep tendon reflexes with evidence of *spasticity;* even conus Babinski and Hofmann signs may occur. Proprioceptive loss is evident, and there may be sensory deficit of cord level and evidence of posterior column dysfunction. There may also be bladder dysfunction of a neurogenic type.

The examination must be thorough in neurologic and musculoskeletal aspects. The fundoscopic examination, cranial nerve examination, and a rectal examination to ascertain sphincter tonus must be included. The objective documentation of the suggestive subjective complaints must be corroberated.

X-ray films of the cervical spine may merely reveal *straightening,* that is, reversal of the lordosis. Ultimately flexion and extension lateral views should be taken to ascertain listhesis and to determine the segment of hypermobility. A

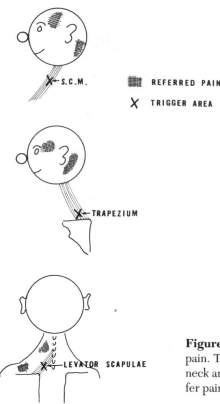

S.C.M.

▓ REFERRED PAIN

X TRIGGER AREA

TRAPEZIUM

LEVATOR SCAPULAE

Figure 6–33. Trigger points and referred pain. Tender areas in various areas of the neck and shoulder, when irritated, can refer pain to distal sites.

CT scan or, preferably, an MRI scan may reveal encroachment into the spinal canal or a herniated disk and deformity of the cord. Dye-invasive studies with CT or a myelogram may also be indicated.

Theories of Mechanism. It has been postulated that in the syndrome of acute central spinal cord injury there has been a contusion of the cord or an acute angulation. The ligamentum flavum may also have been wrinkled or plicated. There may have been momentary occlusion of the arterial supply to the cord (Fig. 6–38).

Treatment. There must be verification as to whether and to which degree there is anatomic abnormality: fracture, dislocation, or fracture-dislocation, and the degree. Precise treatment is best approached by orthopedic or neurosurgic consultation, inasmuch as treatment will vary from total to partial paresis.

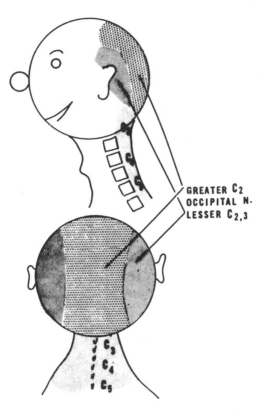

Figure 6–34. Dermatomal distribution of the occipital nerves. The greater occipital and lesser occipital nerves formed from roots C_2, C_3, and C_4 refer pain to the occipital vertex or parietal areas of the head, as depicted by shaded areas.

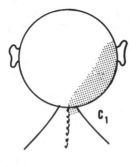

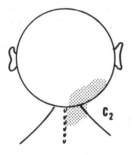

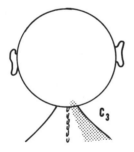

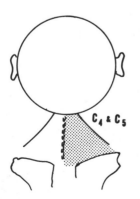

Figure 6–35. Referred zones of root levels. Injection of an irritant into paraspinous areas of the cervical spine (C_1 through C_5) results in pain noted by patients and depicted here in the shaded areas.

Figure 6–36. Greater superior occipital nerve (C_2). The extradural C_2 nerve roots emerge from the cervical spine as shown on right.
C_1—atlas
C_2—axis
C_3—third cervical vertebra
OCC—occiput
M—posterior atlanto-axial membrane
O—odontoid process of axis
PAA—posterior arch of atlas (C-1)
G—ganglion of C_2 nerve
C—capsules of cervical joints
vr—ventral root of C_2
dr—dorsal root of C_2

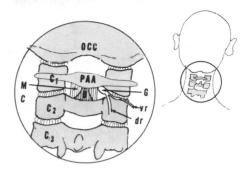

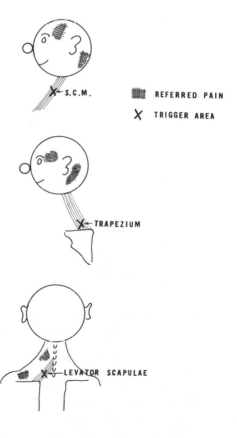

Figure 6–37. Trigger points and referred pain. Tender areas in various areas of the neck and shoulder, when irritated, can refer pain to distal sites.

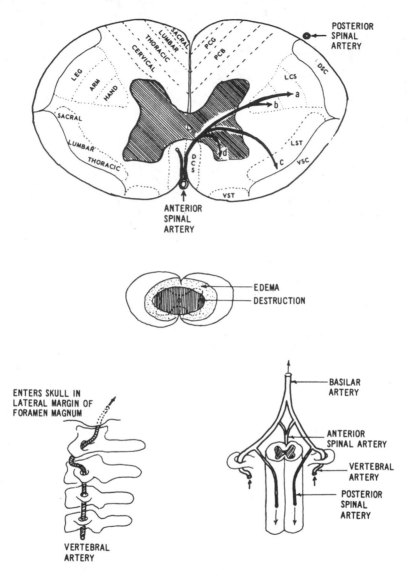

Figure 6–38. Vascular supply to the cervical cord. The arterial circulation that sustains a transient impairment in the syndrome of acute central spinal cord injury is shown. The clinical neurologic symptoms are explained by the cord tracts that sustain the ischemia: a and b supply arm and hand area of lateral corticospinal (pyramidal) tract, c supplies lumbar and thoracic areas of lateral spinothalamic tract, d supplies anterior medical portion of gray matter.

PCG	=	posterior column Goll	LST	=	lateral spinothalamic
PCB	=	posterior column Burdach	VSC	=	ventral spinocerebellar
DCS	=	dorsal spinocerebellar	VST	=	ventral spinothalamic
LCS	=	lateral corticospinal	DSC	=	direct corticospinal

BIBLIOGRAPHY

Barré, MJ: Sur un syndrome sympathique cervical postérieur et sa cause frequente, l'arthrite cervicale. Rev Neur (Paris) 1:1240, 1926.

Dasillajian, JV and Latif, A: Integrated actions and functions of the chief flexors of the elbow: A detailed electromyographic analysis. J Bone Joint Surg 39A:1106, 1957.

Bogduk, N: Headaches and cervical manipulation: Leading articles. Med J Aust 28:65, 1979.

Bogduk, N and Harsland, A: The cervical zygapophyseal joints as a source of neck pain. Spine 13(6):610, 1988.

Bogduk, N: The clinical anatomy of the cervical dorsal rami. Spine 7(4):319, 1982.

Bogduk, N: The anatomy of occipital neuralgia. Clin Exp Neurol 17:167, 1980.

Bosworth, DM: Editorial. J Bone Joint Surg 41-A:16, 1959.

Braaf, MM and Rosner, S: Trauma of the cervical spine as a cause of chronic headache. J Trauma 15:441, 1975.

Braaf, MM and Rosner, S: Whiplash injuries of the neck: Symptoms, diagnosis, treatment and prognosis. New York State J Med 58:1501, 1958.

Brieg, A: Biomechanics of the Central Nervous System. Year Book Publishers, Chicago, 1960.

Buonocore, E, Horstman, T, and Nelson, CL: Cineradiograms of cervical spine in diagnosis of soft tissue injuries. JAMA 198(1):13, 1966.

Cailliet, R: Soft Tissue Pain and Disability, ed 2. FA Davis, Philadelphia, 1988.

Cameron, BM: A,"Whiplash" symposium: Theory critique. Orthopedics 2:127, 1960.

Cammack, KV: Whiplash injuries to the neck. Am J Surg 93:663, 1957.

Campbell, DC and Parsons, EJ: Referred head pain and its concomitants. Nerv Ment Dis 9:554, 1944.

Cheshire, DL: The stability of the cervical spine following the conservative treatment of fractures and fracture-dislocations. Paraplegia 7:193, 1969.

Cloward, RB: Cervical diskography: A contribution to the etiology and mechanism of neck, shoulder and arm pain. Ann Surg 150:1052, 1959.

Chrisman, OD and Gervais, RF: Otological manifestations of the cervical syndrome. Clin Orthop 24:34, 1962.

Colachis, S and Strohm, BB: Cervical traction: Relationship of traction time to varied force with constant angle of ull. Arch Phys Med Rehab 46:815, 1965.

Colachis, S and Strohm, B: Radiographic studies of cervical spine motion in normal subjects: Flexion and hyperextension. Arch Phys Med Rehab 46:753, 1963.

Crowe, H: Injuries to the cervical spine. Presented at the Annual Meeting of the Western Orthopedic Association, San Francisco, 1928.

Crue, BJ: Importance of flexion in cervical traction for radiculitis. USAF Med J 8:375, 1957.

Crue, BJ and Mabie, PD: Conservative treatment of halter traction is acute cervical trauma. West J Surg Obstet Gynecol 68:176, 1960.

Crue, BJ and Todd, EM: The importance of flexion in cervical halter traction. Bull LA Neurol Soc 30:95, 1965.

Fielding, JW: Cineroetgenography of the normal cervical spine. J Bone Joint Surg 39-A:1280, 1957.

Fisher, SV et al: Cervical orthosis effect in cervical spine motion: Roentgenographic and goniometric method of study. Arch Phys Med Rehab 58·109, 1977.

Frykholm, R: Deformities of dural pouches and strictures of dural sheaths in cervical region producing nerve root compression: Contributing to etiology and operative treatment of brachial neuralgia. J Neurol Surg 4:403, 413, 1947.

Greenberg, AD: Atlanto-axial dislocation. Brain 91:655, 1968.

Hall, RF, Stuck, RM, and Hall, OEK: Whiplash: Injury of the cervical spine, II. Orthopedics 109: March 1959.

Harris, JH, Edeiken-Monroe, B, and Kopaniky, DR: A practical classification of acute cervical spine injuries. Orthop Clin North Am 15:30, 1986.

Hohl, M: Soft tissue injuries of the neck in automobile accidents: Factors influencing prognosis. J Bone Joint Surg 56:1675, 1974.

Holdsworth, FW: Fractures, dislocation and fracture dislocation. J Bone Joint Surg 45-B:6, 1963.

Hunter, CR and Mayfield, FH: Role of the upper cervical roots in the production of pain in the head. Am J Surg 78:743, 1949.

Johgkees, LB: Whiplash examination. Laryngoscope 93:113, 1983.

Jones, MD: Cineradiographic studies of abnormalities of the high cervical spine. Arch Surg 94:206, 1967.

Juhl, JH, Miller, SM, and Roberts, GW: Roentgenographic variations in the normal cervical spine. Radiology 78:591, 1962.

Kovacs, A: Subluxation and deformation of the cervical apophyseal joints. Acta Radiol 43:1, 1955.

Krout, RM and Anderson, TP: Role of anterior cervical muscles in production of neck pain. Arch Phys Med Rehabil 47:608, 1956.

Lipow, EG: Whiplash injuries. South Med J 48:1304, 1955.

Louis, H: Surgery of the Spine: Surgical Anatomy and Operative Approaches. Springer-Verlag, Berlin, 1983.

Macnab, I: The "whiplash" syndrome symposium on diseases of the intervertebral disc. Orthop Clin North Am 2:(2)389, 1971.

McGhee, FO: Whiplash: Injuries of the cervical spine, I. Orthopedics 105, March 1959.

MacNamara, RM, O'Brien, MC, and Davidheiser, S: Posttraumatic neck pain: a prospective and follow-up study. Ann Emerg Med 17(9):906, 1988.

Maitland, GD: Vertebral Manipulation, ed 4. Butterworth & Co, London, 1977.

Martinez, JL and Garcia, DJ: A model for whiplash. Journal of Biomechanics 1:23, 1968.

McFarland, JW and Krusen, FA: Use of Sayer head sling in osteoarthritis of cervical portion of spinal column. Arch Phys Med Rehabil 24:263, 1943.

McKeever, DC: The so-called whiplash injury. Orthopedics 2:14, 1960.

Mealy, K, Brennan, H, and Feneron, GCC: Early mobilization of acute whiplash injuries. Br Med J 292:656, 1986.

Mertz, HJ and Patrick, LM: Investigation of the kinematics and kinetics of whiplash. In Stapp, JP: Medical Aspects of Safety Seat Belt Conference. October 1967.

Munro, R: Treatment of fractures and dislocations of the cervical spine. N Engl J Med 264:573, 1961.

Panjabi, MD and White, AA: Clinical Biomechanics of the Spine. JB Lippincott, Philadelphia, 1978.

Reynolds, GG, Pavot, AP and Kendrick, MM: Electromyographic evaluation of patients with post-traumatic cervical pain. Arch Phys Med Rehabil. 170, March 1968.

Saternus, KS: The mechanics of whiplash injury of the cervical spine (German-English abstract). Z Rechtsmed 88:1, 1982.

Schneider, RC and Crosby, EC: Vascular insufficiency of brainstem and spinal cord in spinal trauma. Neurology 9:643, 56, 1960.

Schneider, RC and Schemm, GW: Vertebral artery insufficiency in acute and chronic spinal trauma, with reference to the syndrome of acute central cervical spinal cord injury. J Neurosurg 18:348, 1961.

Schutt, CH and Dohan, EC: Neck injuries to women in auto accidents. JAMA 206:2689, 1968.

Selecki, BR: Whiplash: A specialist's view. Australian Family Physician 13:243, 1984.

Severy, DM, Mathewson, JH, and Bechtol, CO: Controlled automobile rearend collision: An investigation of related engineering and medical phenomena. CMAJA 11:727, 1955.

Stedman's Medical Dictionary, ed 23. Williams & Wilkins, Baltimore, 1976.

Su, HC and Su, RK: Treatment of whiplash injuries with acupuncture. Clin J Pain 4:233, 1988.

Tomita, K, Tsuchiya, H, and Nomua, S: Dynamic entrapment of the vertebral artery by the nerve branch: A new etiology for transient cervical vertigo. Neuro-orthopedics 4:36, 1987.

Travell, J and Simons, D: Myofascial pain and dysfunction, the trigger point manual. Williams & Wilkins, Baltimore, 1983.

Trevor-Jones, R: Osteo-arthritis of the paravertebral joints of the second and third cervical vertebrae as a cause of occipital headaches. S Afr Med J 392:(394)30, 1964.

Warfield, CA, et al: Epidural steroid injection as a treatment for cervical radiculitis Clin J Pain 4:201, 1988.

Waylonis, GW: Electromyographic findings in chronic cervical radicular syndromes. Arch Phys Med Rehabil 407, July 1968.

White, AA and Panjabi, MM: Clinical Biomechanics of the Spine. JB Lippincott, Philadelphia, 1978.

Yoss, RE, et al: Significance of symptoms and signs in localization of involved root in cervical disc protrusion. Neurology 7(10)673, 1957.

The Revolt Against "Whiplash." The Defense Research Institute, Syracuse, 1958.

CHAPTER 7

Cervical Disk Disease in the Production of Pain and Disability

For years it has been accepted that increased internal pressure within an intervertebral disk could evoke pain (Hirsch). Initially, the innervation of the intervertebral disk for the transmission of painful stimuli was not clarified nor even accepted (Roofe). There were, and still are, investigators and clinicians who deny the presence of any unmyelinated nerves capable of transmitting painful stimuli within the disk. No nerve endings have been identified within the nucleus or within the inner annular fibers of an intact normal disk.

Recently nerve fiber endings have been identified within the outer annular layers of the intervertebral disk capable of transmitting painful sensations. Whether these endings are actually from nerves penetrating the annulus or are nerve endings within the longitudinal ligaments has not been clarified. They are, however, considered to be a neurologic basis for *diskogenic pain*.

These nerve endings are considered to be the terminus of the sinuvertebral nerves of Luschka and contain both somatic and sympathetic nerve fibers. These have been discussed in Chapter 1. These nerve endings are also similar to the nerve ending supplying the anterior and posterior longitudinal ligaments.

Pain originating in the neck and felt in the neck or shoulder, arm, hand, or fingers *from* the neck usually results from irritation of the cervical nerve roots within the region of the intervertebral foramina.

Initiation of pain can be considered a result of encroachment on the nerve within the foramen from tissues forming the foramen borders. The tissues forming the foramina (as discussed in Chapter 1) are as follows:

1. Anteriorly: the posterior aspects of the vertebral bodies, the posterior longitudinal ligament, and the posterior annular fibers of the disk

2. Superiorly and inferiorly: the pedicles of the posterior neural canal complex
3. Posteriorly: the facets and their capsules (zygapophyseal joints) and the ligamentum flavum

The size of the foramina is dependent upon the integrity of the intervertebral disk, which separates the vertebral bodies and thus separates the pedicles and the posterior facet joints. The internal pressure within the disk makes taut (stiffens) the outer annular fibers and the longitudinal ligaments.

Normal neck movement modifies the size and shape of the foramina. Flexion of the cervical spine *opens* the foramina, and extension *closes* them. Rotation and lateral flexion open them on the convex borders and close them on the concave side toward which they flex or rotate. These are normal physiologic changes that do not normally encroach upon the nerve roots or their dural sheaths (see Chapter 1).

Of the numerous tissues within the cervical spine to which pain production and disability can be attributed, the disk has been given major importance. There are many clinicians who would refute this predominence, but the pathologic disk is a cause of major significance and must be thoroughly evaluated.

The disk is involved in both acute and chronic pathology. The former implies herniation involving the neural contents of the foramen, and the latter, its role in degenerative disk disease.

The intervertebral disk must also be evaluated as causing neck pain and arm, hand, and finger *referred* pain. Encroachment from the disk upon the nerve supply to these two regions—the neck and the upper extremity—requires clarification. The exact tissue component of the disk, the nucleus or the annulus, also needs to be understood.

As in all neuromusculoskeletal painful syndromes, there must be a clarification of taxonomy. There must be a clear understanding of diagnostic terms. *Slipped disk, ruptured disk, bulging disk, herniated disk,* and so forth are terms used with little or no clear understanding of the exact pathology or of the relationship of the pathologic tissue change with the clinical symptomatology.

Much of the research of diskogenic pathology concerned the lumbosacral spine, but there is increasing study to clarify similar changes in the disk tissues of the cervical spine. The anatomic, chemical, nutritional, reparative, and degenerative changes of one are similar to those of the other. The resultant pathology is also not dissimilar.

It must be remembered that the contents of the spinal canal in the lumbosacral spine are significantly different from those within the cervical spine. In the former are located the nerve roots of the cauda equina, whereas in the cervical spine is contained the spinal cord as well as the nerve roots. There is also a structural difference between the cervical disk and the lumbar disk (Figs. 7–1 to 7–3).

It must also be remembered that radiculopathy —that is, referred pain from nerve root entrapment— occurs in the upper cervical spine (occiput-atlas-

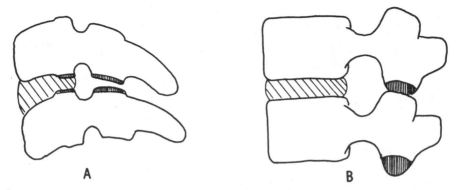

Figure 7–1. Comparative lateral views of cervical and lumbar functional units. *(A)* Cervical spine: five joints; disk, paired intervertebral arthroses, and posterior articulations. *(B)* Lumbar spine: three joints; disk, and paired posterior articulations.

axis), wherein there is no disk.

Recent discussion regarding *internal disk herniation,* wherein the nucleus herniated within the confines of the annulus as opposed to outside the annular region, has concerned primarily the lumbar disk. Such a similar pathologic change undoubtedly occurs in the cervical disk.

Diskography has shed light upon the symptoms caused by changes of the nucleus and annulus and pressure changes within the intervertebral disk (Cloward, 1959). Recent magnetic resonance imaging (MRI) studies, which re-

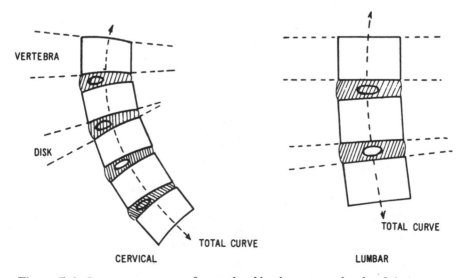

Figure 7–2. Comparative curves of cervical and lumbar spine: related to disk shapes.

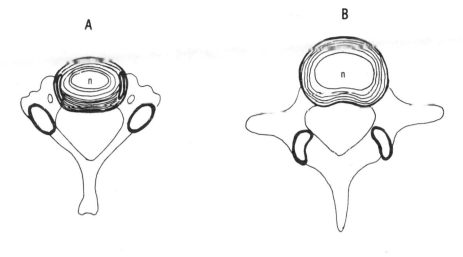

Figure 7–3. Vertebral bodies of cervical and lumbar region: comparing joints and disks. (*A*) Cervical segment. Five joints (including intervertebral articulations). Cervical disks: anterior height 2–3 times greater than posterior. Nucleus, anterior position. Annulus, thicker posterior. (*B*) Lumbar segment. Three joints. Lumbar disks: anterior height slightly greater than posterior. Nucleus, middle position. Annulus, symmetrical.

veal the internal structural changes within the intervertebral disk as related to the symptoms claimed by the patient, have also clarified many of these factors.

Increase of internal pressure in a defective disk is known to cause pain to the patient both in the vicinity of the interscapular area and in the neck region. Mere touch of the outer annular fibers has also caused this local and referred pain.

Pain in the interscapular region has been attributed to mechanical trauma to the anterior longitudinal ligament and the anterior outer annular fibers in the process of performing a diskogram (Fig. 7–4). The area of referred pain in the interscapular area can also be eliminated by local injection of an anesthetic agent (Michelsen and Mixter) into the referral area (Elliot and Kremer). The referral area of pain in the interscapular area reveals hyperirritability on an electromyogram (EMG) examination of the area, but there is no evidence of nerve root damage (Wedell and others).

The motor nerve supply to the muscles of the interscapular region is as follows:

C_3 to C_4: Levator scapulae muscles
C_5: Rhomboid muscles

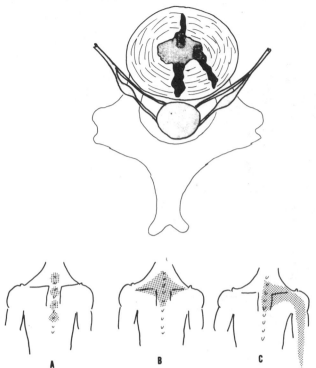

Figure 7–4. Referral sites of pain elicited by intranuclear diskograms. (A) Irritation of the anterior portion of the disk refers pain to the interscapular midline. (B) Posterior nucleus protrusion refers pain as depicted. (C) Posterior lateral protrusion into the region of the intervertebral foramen causes interscapular pain plus arm radicular pain in the distribution of the nerve root dermatome.

C_5 to C_6: Supraspinatus muscles
C_6 to C_7: Latissmus dorsi muscles

The dermatomal pattern of the interscapular region is by T_7 roots and thus not from the cervical spine roots.

It appears that this referred pain is muscular (myotomal) and not neurogenic, that is, not referred from a single nerve root. Frykholm (1951) reproduced scapular pain when he irritated the ventral (motor) nerve root intradurally. He stated that the pain was found to be "more deeply situated and referred to the proximal part of the limb and shoulder girdle . . . and tender to pressure." The sensation so noted "was different from the pain elicited by stimulation of the sensory nerve roots." In correlating these clinical findings it is difficult to ascertain whether this interscapular pain is essentially diskogenic or neurogenic, yet the pain can be reproduced by mere involvement of the outer annular fibers and not necessarily from irritation of either sensory or motor nerve root.

New terminology, therefore, evolves: *diskogenic, myalgic,* or *neuralgic.* The area of referral also is differentiated into *dermatomal* and *sclerotomal.* The tissue site of pain within and from the cervical spine functional unit can come from any of the soft tissues, among which the intervertebral disk is a component.

NEUROGENIC RADICULAR PAIN

The relationship of the nerve root to the intervertebral disk as the root emerges through the foramen has been documented. The difference in is anatomic proximity of the lumbar to the cervical region is noted in Figure 7–5.

Within the cervical functional unit the nerve root is protected from trauma by the presence of the posterior longitudinal ligament covering the posterior aspect of the disk, which in turn is double-layered in that area. The nucleus of the cervical disk is also not central, as it is in the lumbar spine but, rather, is anteriorly placed and therefore is surrounded posteriorly by numerous layers (sheaths) of annular fibers. There are also the uncovertebral joints (the prominences of von Luschka) situated between the nucleus and the nerve roots bilaterally.

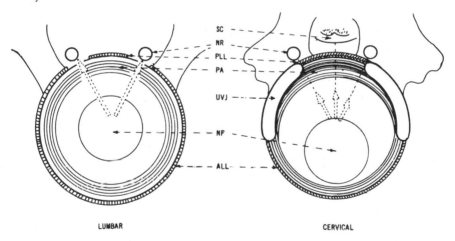

LUMBAR   CERVICAL

Figure 7–5. Comparison of lumbar and cervical disk containers. The lumbar region has an incomplete posterior longitudinal ligament, PLL, a thin layer posteriorly of the annulus fibrosus, PA, and thus a relatively exposed nerve root, NR. Arrows show the routes by which herniation of the nucleus can approach the nerve roots. The nucleus pulposus, NP, is centrally located. The cervical region has a posterior longitudinal ligament, PLL, spanning the entire posterior portion of the vertebral body, a double-layered ligament. The posterior portion of the annulus, PA, is broader and firmer. The nerve root, NR, is partially protected by the interposed uncovertebral joints of von Luschka, UVJ, and the anterior position of the nucleus, NP, places it far from the nerve roots and the spinal cord, SP, from the protruding disk material.

There are aging changes within the disk that also influence the type and severity of disk herniation, internal or external. When there have been annular tears or disruption, healing of the collagen is mostly by invasion of connective tissue, causing a fibrous *scarring*. These healing tissue changes are similar to healing of cartilage, which is by fibrocartilagenous tissue rather than by the original pure collagen fibers. This fibrous repair tissue has neither the hydrodynamic potential nor the ability to react to outer stresses that normally stiffen the disk.

Whether the symptoms claimed by the patient are directly related to the disruption of the disk is an enigma faced by any clinicians. There are those who claim that neck and arm pain are rarely caused by disk pathology, but others claim that any neck and arm radiating pain is the result of a nerve being impacted by a disk protrusion. Somewhere between these two extremes undoubtedly lies the truth.

Herniation of the nucleus within the annulus can occur (Fig. 7–6). This inner herniation will cause neck pain and possibly some upper extremity pain if there is some concomitant bulging of the annulus (Fig. 7–7). The annulus bulges because of the internal pressure of the nucleus through annular tears which permit the nucleus to protrude outward.

Protrusion of the annulus is possible in numerous directions (Fig. 7–8). If the annular protrusion is directly posterior, only the posterior longitudinal ligament can cause neck and arm pain. If the annulus bulges posterior laterally, it is possible for the pressure upon the specific nerve root of that level *and* the posterior longitudinal ligament to induce pain.

The posterior lateral protrusion of the annulus places the nerve root under tension and may result in radicular pain in the region of the dermatome. It may also cause radiation of pain into a muscle group (myotome) region via irritation of the motor nerve root, as has been postulated by Frykholm (1951). Both areas of radiation, dermatome and myotome, are similar because they are innervated by similar nerve roots.

Clinically the patient presents (history) with pain in the neck, limited neck range of passive and active of motion, and subjective sensation of pain, numbness, or tingling in the dermatomal region. The cause of the pain is also to be ascertained from the history as to external trauma, prolonged abnormal posture, and severe prolonged emotional tension. The external trauma may be an auto-versus-auto accident, a fall, a slip, a manipulation, and so forth.

The extent of the external trauma must be clarified as to (1) postulated force of impact, (2) awareness of the patient at the moment of impact, (3) the direction of the face and neck the moment of impact, (4) the status of the patient's neck and general health before the accident.

The examination reveals (1) guarding by the patient when moving the neck, (2) assuming a protective neck posture, such as holding the head and neck to one side, avoiding extension, and so forth, (3) reproducing the pain initiated by the patient's active motion of the neck, and (4) confirming by specific motion and position what the patient's initial restriction implies.

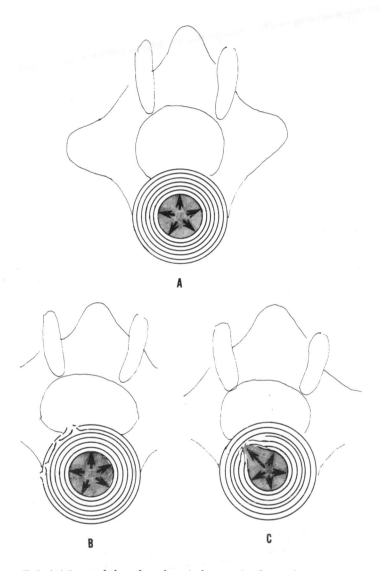

Figure 7–6. (A) Intact disk and nucleus (schematic). The nucleus is intact and its intrinsic forces (arrows) are expended equally in all directions. (B) Intact nucleus with disruption of outer annular fibers (schematic). The outer annular fibers have been disrupted, but there are sufficient annular fibers to contain the intact nucleus. The arrows indicate intrinsic forces within the nucleus but no annulus bulging. (C) Intact annulus (no bulge) but extrusion of the nucleus (schematic). The nucleus has extruded from the inner annular fibers, but there are sufficient intact outer annular fibers to prevent significant extrusion of the annulus into the canals.

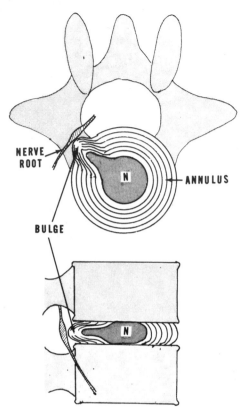

NERVE ROOT

N

ANNULUS

BULGE

N

Figure 7–7. Central extrusion of nucleus, causing external extrusion of annulus. *(Top)* Internal extrusion *(rupture)* of the nucleus in a posterior lateral direction. The weakened annular fibers permit external extrusion of the overlaying annular fibers, causing pressure upon the nerve root. *(bottom)*.

Passively extending the neck may initiate the pain, as may flexion, lateral flexion, and/or rotation. These motions and their relationship to the foramina have been discussed in Chapter 1. Extension narrows the foramina; flexion opens them but also places traction on the nerve root. Rotation or lateral flexion closes the foramina on the side to which rotation is assumed and opens the foramina on the side away from which rotation occurs.

An aspect of the examination, frequently not performed, is digital palpation of the foramina on either side of the neck, which irritates the entrapped nerve root and causes local pain and tenderness or even radiation of pain in the dermatomal direction claimed by the patient.

Limitation of neck range of motion must be directed to differentiate occipital cervical motion (occiput-atlas-axis) from cervical spine (C-3 to C-7) motion. Specific localization by manual mobilization of, for instance, C-5 to 6 or C-6–7 is difficult, if not impossible. The specific site of limitation of the lower segment of the cervical spine as to a segmental level is made by (1) limited cervical motion in flexion, extension, or rotation-lateral flexion; (2) subjective localization, by the patient, as to *where* the sensation radiates; and (3) direct localization of the precise foramen by direct manual palpation of the neck.

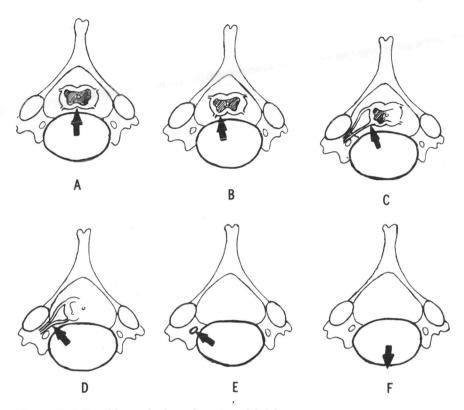

Figure 7–8. Possible results from direction of disk herniation.
A = dorsomedial herniation may cause bilaternal cord compression.
B = paramedical herniation: unilaternal cord compression.
C = dorsolateral protrusion: unilaternal cord and nerve root compression.
D = intraforaminal protrusion: radicle nerve root compression.
E = laternal protrusion: vertebral artery and nerve compression.
F = ventral protrusion causes no nerve root, cord, or vertebral artery compression.

A precise central disk internal nucleus herniation with an annulus bulge can be confirmed by CT scanning or MRI. These tests reveal the presence of and the location of the bulging disk. It must always be remembered, however, that the *diagnosis of a bulging disk is made clinically by history and physical examination and confirmed by* CT or MRI. Never should a diagnosis be made merely upon the interpretation of these tests.

Nerve root entrapment can occur posteriorly by nerve pressure from an osteophyte rather than anteriorly by a bulging annulus. Here the diagnosis is also a clinical diagnosis and is confirmable by CT or MRI.

EXTRUDED NUCLEUS PULPOSUS

Extrusion of the nucleus from the annular confines is a *true* disk herniation. This condition is *extrusion of the nucleus* and must be labeled as such. The clinical picture may be similar to an annular bulge, and often the differentiation can be made only by CT scan, MRI, or surgical intervention.

There are essentially six possible directions of disk herniation, as shown in Figure 7–6. The possibility of central herniation with cord compression must always be kept in mind, and upper motor neuron testing be part of every examination.

LOCALIZATION OF ROOT LEVEL
BY CLINICAL EXAMINATION

Precise cervical disk level with accurate root localization may be possible by myelography, MRI, CT scanning, or EMG, but a reasonably accurate clinical localization is possible.

Clinical localization is suggested by (1) subjective sensory localization from the history—where the patient feels hyperesthesia, paresthesia, or hypoesthesia; (2) objective localization during the examination from light touch such as a scratch from a pin or cotton; and (3) subjective motor weakness claimed by the patient during activities of daily living; which can be confirmed by (4) objective muscle testing and (5) deep tendon reflex changes.

Subjective sensation localization is suggestive but rarely accurate. A dermatomal complaint of aching or tenderness is difficult to differentiate from one of a sclerotomal region. The sensation of *spasm* experienced by the patient is also usually too diffuse and vague to be of value in localizing a root level.

Specific nerve root localization is also made inexact (Benini) because there are many anatomic variations in nerve roots that make exact localization precarious. These anatomic variations vary from peripheral anastomosis of the ulnar and median nerves, anastomosis in the brachial plexus, variations of specific motor units receiving their supply from a specific nerve root(s), and the fact that sensation now is known to be transmitted via a motor nerve root in direct contradiction to the Bell-Magendie law.

As has been stated, neurogenic pain must be differentiated from discogenic pain (see Fig. 7–4). Neurogenic pain is felt only when the disk protrusion (nucleus or annulus) encroaches upon the nerve root. When subjected to traction, the nerve root normally responds with painful sensory input to the patient.

Pain more distal in radiation is dermatomal in distribution, whereas pain proximal to the interscapular area is more likely from posterior primary division radicular pain. Radicular pain varies from a deep aching sensation to a sharp pain superimposed upon a dull ache. It is not uncommon for radicular pain of an aching nature to be felt proximally and a paresthesia or sensation of numbness to be felt distally. The possibility of motor nerve sensation (via the myotomal distribution) explains, in part, the sensation of pain and the presence of tenderness in distal muscles of the upper extremity.

As stated in Chapter 1, neck flexion causes upward movement of the nerve within the spinal canal and thus increases root tension within the root canals but with no increased tension of the dural root pouches (these unfold). The roots are firmly fixed at the outer rim of the intervertebral foramina (Fig. 7–9). The intrathecal (intraspinal) roots move about these points of fibrous attachment.

When the head and neck is extended, the roots ascend within the foraminal gutter; that is, the roots migrate superiorly in the foramen. In the flexed position they descend; that is, they migrate caudally. The nerve roots normally are placed under more tension upon flexion. The dural sac unfolds and actually elongates during neck flexion. There is adequate physiologic elongation of the dural sac so as to not encroach upon the enclosed nerve roots.

If there is an increase in the tension of the nerve root and its dural sac from a protruding disk, the elongation of the dural sheath is thwarted and compression of the dural contents occurs. The dentate ligament which supports the cord within the spinal canal connects to the dural sac. In cervical flexion the canal elongates, as does the enclosed cord. The dentate ligaments, being inelastic and

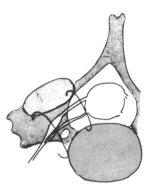

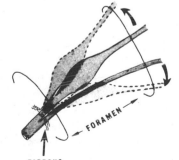

Figure 7–9. Movement of nerve roots about their point of attachment. The nerve roots are anchored at the outer area of the foramen. As the intradural nerves move, cranially during flexion and caudally during neck extension, the roots angle about their fibrous attachment (point of fixation). This explains increased nerve tension during these movements.

FORAMEN

FIBROUS
ATTACHMENT

anchored to the bony canal and the cord dura, exert traction upon the cord. The cord, thus laterally distracted, narrows in its anterior posterior width. The roots also are thus elongated at their fila. When the cord is stretched in neck flexion, so are the nerve roots stretched.

A radicular sensation occurs from neck flexion when there has been a protrusion of a disk into the nerve root gutter, inasmuch as the root is more taut and less elastic.

Extension of the neck narrows the length of the spinal canal and simultaneously closes the foramina. If the nerve root and its dura have been encroached upon with resultant inflammation, this motion of the neck may also cause radiculopathy. Clinically either movement, flexion or extension, reproduces the radicular painful sensation claimed by the patient and may be reproduced during the examination.

In differentiating radiculopathy from a protruding disk versus encroachment upon the nerve root from an osteophytic spur, this aspect of foraminal opening and closing with movement of the nerve root and its dura must be kept in mind. As a general rule, extension (closing the foramina) more probably encroaches upon a nerve root in cervical spondylosis, and flexion probably distracts the nerve root in the presence of a disk herniation.

Changes seen on x-ray film, CT scan, or MRI only enhance the explanation but do not eliminate the explanation engendered by the examination and reproduction of pain by specific motions.

Localization of a dermatome is more specific in the levels of C_5, C_6, C_7, or C_8 because these refer to more specific finger distributions. Reference to the upper arm or the forearm is less precise. In the hand, C_5 to C_6 roots refer mostly to the thumb, C_6 to the middle finger, and C_7 to C_8 to the little finger (Fig. 7–10). The average astute examiner will minimize the accuracy of either subjective or objective localization.

There are three clinical tests that have proven effective in confirming that there is radiculitis of cervical root origin. These tests are the Spurling neck compression test (Fig. 7–11), the axial manual traction test, and the arm abduction test (Fig. 7–12) (Viikari-Juntura and others).

The neck compression test is performed by having the patient seated with the head laterally flexed and rotated *to* the side of the radicular pain. Pressure is exerted downward upon the head. This maneuver actually closes the foramina on the side toward which the pain is felt, and the downward compression further closes the foramina and compresses the disk, thus increasing its protrusion.

The manual traction test merely elongated the cervical spine with a resultant distraction of each functional unit and a decrease in the lordosis. Relief, albeit momentary, indicates that there is nerve root compression. The overhead arm abduction test is performed by placing the patient in a seated position and elevating the affected arm over the head. This decreases the traction upon the involved nerve root.

Positive results of these three tests confirm that there is nerve root com-

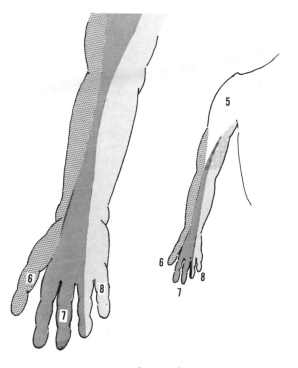

Figure 7–10. Dermatomes of cervical nerve roots C_5 to C_8.

pression within the foramina, conceivably but not proven by a herniated disk. There is *no* specific root level localization by these three maneuvers, only a confirmation that nerve root compression occurs at the foraminal levels.

Muscle testing (myotome) is far more precise in localizing a specific root level. Weakness of the upper arm external rotator is specific for C_5 to C_6; the deltoid, C_5; the wrist extensor, C_6; the brachialis, C_6; and the triceps, C_7.

All muscle tests should be performed with the patient in a position to isolate the muscle being tested. Other actions of that muscle group or of other muscles with different nerve supply must be minimized. For instance, the deltoid muscle is best tested with the patient in the standing position. The biceps tendon reflex is best tested with the patient seated, and the triceps tendon reflex with the patient in the supine position.

Testing the triceps in the supine position with the arm extending toward the ceiling facilitates isolating the triceps muscle and thus tests C_7 root (Fig. 7–13). The external rotators (C_5 to C_6) are also best tested in the supine position (Fig. 7–14).

Testing C_8 implies testing the strength of the finger intrinsics. This testing can best be done with the patient in the seated position facing the examiner, who can also detect atrophy if present.

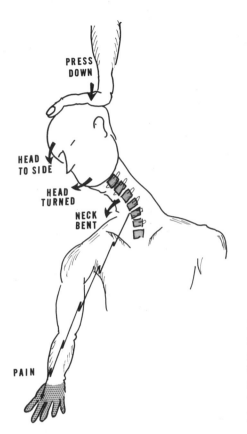

Figure 7–11. Neck compression test for radiculitis. With the patient seated and the head turned and laterally flexed to the side of the radiculitis, there is then downward compression upon the head. A *positive* test result reproduces the radicular symptoms.

The deep tendon reflexes are done in the routine neurologic manner and are reliable in denoting a specific root level.

The brachioradialis reflex (C_6) is tested with the forearm in a neutral mid-position of pronation and supination with the elbow flexed (Fig. 7–15). In the presence of a root lesion (C_6) there may be elicited a finger flexion response and but no elbow flexion. This finding is termed *inversion* of the radial reflex.

The test for the pronator reflex (C_7) is performed in a similar manner to that for the brachioradialis reflex, but the hammer impact is to the side of, and not down upon, the radius. For this reflex test the forearm must be flexed at the elbow and held in a neutral pronation supination position (Fig. 7–16).

The response of the pronator tendon reflex is primarily that of reflex pronation of the forearm. Upon the proper hammer impact, finger flexion or elbow flexion rather than forearm pronation indicates a different root level. A clinical significance of this pronator tendon reflex is that it is sufficiently sensitive to be hyperactive in the presence of cord involvement, revealing an upper motor neuron response.

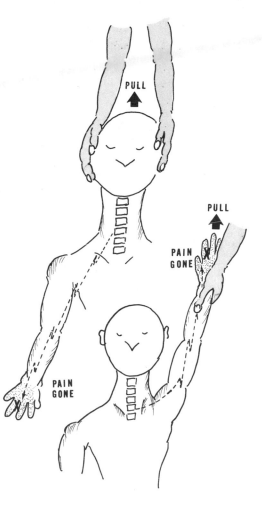

Figure 7–12. Manual traction and arm abduction test for cervical radiculitis. Upper figure depicts manual action upon the head. If there is disappearance or diminution of radicular symptoms, the test result is positive. Lower figure depicts elevation above the head of the arm of the side of the radiculitis. Disappearance of symptoms is a positive test result.

Root Level Summary

Figures 7–17 to 7–20 illustrate the characteristics that localize the specific root level.

A reasonably accurate localization of the root level can, therefore, be made by a careful clinical examination. The subjective sensory levels claimed by the patient in the history are suggestive of a specific level. Impairment of ADL from loss of sensation claimed by the patient is also indicative. Objective sensory testing with cotton touch, light finger touch, pin prick, or pinwheel aid confirmation. However, due to overlap and indistinct area mapping, the sensory testing is considered woefully inaccurate.

Motor testing and tendon reflex testing for root localization are more accurate and, even though there is overlapping and multiple nerve roots to many

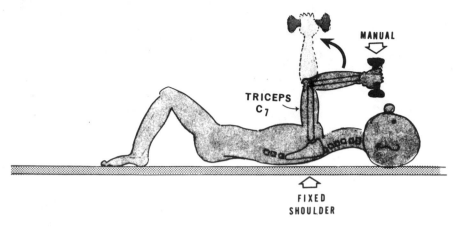

Figure 7–13. Muscle examination of triceps (C_7). With patient supine and arm held vertically, the triceps can more easily be tested for strength and for endurance. In this position the scapular muscles are fixed, allowing the triceps to be isolated (C_7). Fatigue may indicate a C_7 lesion when a single effort fails to reveal weakness.

muscle groups, a careful test helps localize the specific root level. Eliciting fatigue of a muscle contraction, as well as demonstrating local muscle group weakness, may also indicate nerve root impairment in early disk disease.

Accurate tendon reflex testing also indicates nerve root level.

That a specific nerve root is involved does not, per se, implicate a herniated, extruded, or bulging intervertebral disk as the causative factor. Only a thorough history, exhaustive physical and neurologic examinations, and proper correlation with confirmatory tests (CT scanning, MRI, EMG, cortical evoked potential) give an accurate pathophysiologic diagnosis.

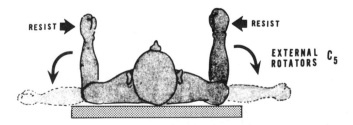

Figure 7–14. External rotator testing to test the supraspinatus and infraspinatus muscles and to determine integrity of the C_5 root. The patient is best placed in the supine position with arms held at the side. Resisting the forearm as the patient attempts external rotation facilitates this muscle examination.

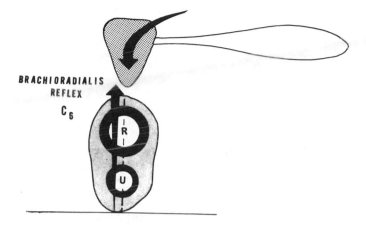

Figure 7–15. Brachioradialis reflex test. With the forearm gently supported and neutral between pronation and supination, a gentle tap on the distal radius or the styloid (attachment of the brachioradialis muscle) will cause reflex flexion of the elbow. The fingers may also flex but are not a part of the brachioradialis reflex. Finger flexion with no elbow flexion—an *inversion*—implies a C_6 lesion.

Figure 7–16. Pronator reflex test. With the forearm slightly pronated (10 to 15°) and lightly supported, the reflex hammer is swung gently to tap the radial styloid on the volar surface. This reflex stretches the pronator teres and causes the forearm to pronate. This reflex is mediated via the C_7 root.

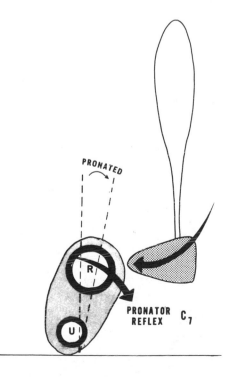

Root	Referred Pain	Paresthesia	Weakness	Reflex
C_5	shoulder and upper arm	none in digit	shoulder	biceps
C_6*	radial aspect forearm	thumb ·	biceps brachioradialis wrist extensor	biceps
C_7†	dorsal aspect forearm	index and middle fingers	triceps	triceps
C_8††	ulnar aspect forearm	ring and little fingers	finger intrinsics	triceps

Figure 7–17. Specific root level.

Electrophysiological studies are now well established in localizing which nerve root is involved (Shea and colleagues). There remains controversy, however, as to whether the peripheral neuropathy is of a nerve root lesion, a brachial plexus lesion, or a peripheral neuropathy (Khan and others).

In studying F wave measurements, these have been found valuable in lumbar radiculopathy but not in lesion of the cervical roots other than C_8 to T_1. Al-

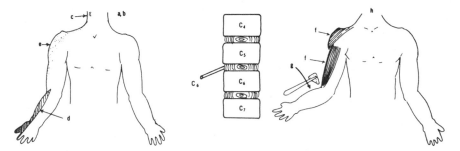

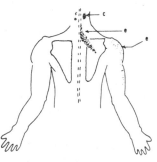

Figure 7–18. Sixth cervical nerve root irritation.

a = Neck rigidity. Limited extension and rotation to the right.

b = Pain and paresthesia aggravated by coughing and sneezing.

c = Tenderness over exit of C_6 nerve root.

d = Paresthesia and hypasthesia of thumb and some of index finger (from history and physical examination).

e = Subjective pain and tenderness over deltoid and rhomboid muscle areas.

f = Weakness of deltoid and biceps muscles.

g = Depressed biceps jerk.

h = X-ray studies equivocal.

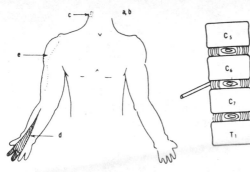
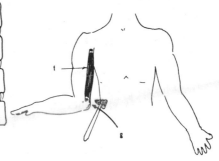

Figure 7–19. Seventh cervical nerve root irritation.

a = Neck rigidity. Limited extension and rotation to the involved side.

b = Pain and paresthesia aggravated by coughing and sneezing.

c = Tenderness over exit of C_7.

d = Paresthesia and hypesthesia of index and middle finger.

e = Subjective deep pain and tenderness of dorsolateral upper arm and superiomedial angle of scapula.

f = Weakness of triceps (also possible biceps).

g = Depressed triceps jerk

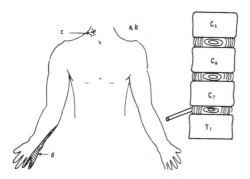
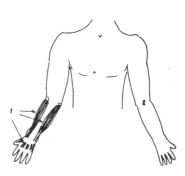

Figure 7–20. Eighth cervical nerve root irritation.

a = Neck rigidity. Limited extension and rotation to the involved side.

b = Pain and paresthesia aggravated by coughing and sneezing.

c = Tenderness over exit of C_8.

d = Paresthesia and hypesthesia of inner forearm and little finger.

e = Subjective deep pain and tenderness from scapula down inner side of upper arm, inner forearm, to little finger.

f = Weakness of hand muscles.

g = No reflex changes.

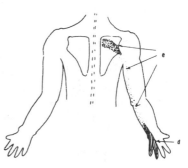

143

though these electrophysiologic studies are, as yet, considered imprecise as to root levels (Khan), they may be useful in screening prior to myelography, or in CT scanning when there is the possibility of surgery.

TREATMENT OF THE CERVICAL HERNIATED DISK

There is consensus among experienced clinicians treating the herniated cervical disk to consider every conservative nonsurgical therapeutic approach before considering surgical intervention.

Barrie Vernon-Roberts categorically states that "the lower discs, commonly C7, tend to be affected and neurological deficit may be evident. The condition usually resolves spontaneously within a few days and conservative treatment only is required in most instances . . . but operative intervention may be required to remove the pressure on the neural tissues." This appears to be the accepted axiom pertaining to treatment of a herniated disk, with certain aspects requiring edification.

When there is *objective* evidence of pressure on neural tissues, essentially pressure upon the nerve root(s), from a disk annular or nuclear herniation, the extent of the nerve impairment must be ascertained.

Pressure from a central disk herniation upon the spinal cord with resultant upper motor neuron signs and symptoms—positive Babinski or Hoffman test results, hyperactive deep tendon reflexes of upper and/or lower extremity, a positive Lermittes's sign, neurogenic bowel and/or bladder dysfunction—by confirmatory tests signals urgent or even emergency surgical intervention. The neurologic signs confirmed by abnormal CT, MRI, myelogram, or cortical evoked potential test indicate a surgical urgency.

In the presence of nerve root impairment the decision to consider surgical intervention resides upon documenting objective neurologic signs that mean functional impairment for the patient. The emphasis of this axiom is on the term *functional*. Functional impairment means that persistence of an objective neurologic deficit may cause impairment or disability that is not tolerable or acceptable for the patient.

Because the usual cervical disk herniation occurs in the foraminal space of C_6, C_7, or C_8 roots, loss of sensation in the hand and fingers is in the distribution of the first (index) finger, middle fingers, or little finger. The first fingers are necessary for prehension and fine dexterity. A loss of C_6, for instance, may impair writing, threading a needle, buttoning buttons, typing, and so forth and thus, if persistent or permanent, may create severe functional loss in ADL or professional pursuit.

It is an accepted neurologic sequela that persistent pressure upon a nerve root of three-months' duration may not recover when the pressure is relieved. Careful monitoring of the patient with weekly objective tests must be done to ascertain the persistence, aggravation, or the amelioration of the sensory deficit before blandly adhering to the dictum *no surgery for three months*.

Loss of sensation of the C_7 or C_8 dermatome may not be of as great a serious functional impairment. Only a careful assessment by an occupational therapist in the ADL or evaluation of the performance requirement of a special occupation will inform both the physician and the patient on the significance of the neural loss.

Loss of the C_5 dermatome may also impair function if there is loss of sensation in the thumb. This dermatome is considered to be in the deltoid region, and loss of sensation there would not usually be a severe functional loss.

Myotomal loss is also to be determined from a functional basis. A C_7 lesion may impair triceps strength, which may not handicap a person unless there is a need to push-pull in his or her daily occupation (push-up in exercise, and so forth), in which case a handicap occurs.

A C_6 lesion may weaken the wrist extensors and cause a functional disability, and a C_5 lesion may weaken the thumb flexors as well as partially weaken elbow flexion external or shoulder rotation. The external rotators are innervated

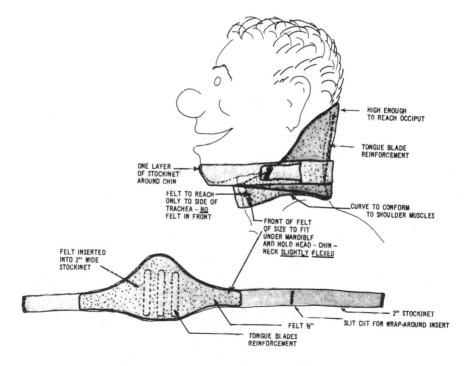

Figure 7–21. Felt collar recommended for occipitoma vical restriction

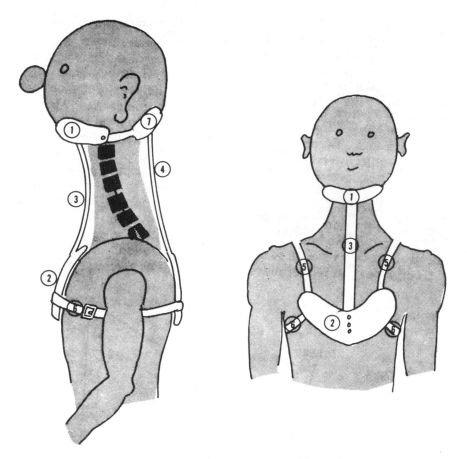

Figure 7-22. SOMI cervical orthosis. This brace is molded with plastic and metal to conform to portions of the head and the shoulders. It fits under the chin (1) and holds the submandibular portion in place by a bent vertical bar (3) arising from a pad against the sternum (2). A posterior bar (4) supports the occipital pad (7). Straps (5,6,7) fasten the brace to body and pass over the shoulders.

by C_5 to C_6 and thus may only fatigue rather than be paretic in a single nerve lesion.

The summary of evaluating the acceptance by the patient of neural loss is a careful functional test once the specific nerve root level is determined by clinical examination and confirmed by EMG examination.

It must be reiterated that a time factor enters the equation: nerve loss, whether sensory or motor/ for a period of time / preferrably less than three months / that is not progressive / acceptable for daily activities. This is a guideline, but the nerve loss must be monitored and discussed with the patient before surgery is contemplated and recommended.

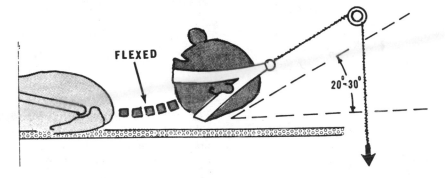

Figure 7–23. Cervical traction applied to the supine patient, causing cervical spine flexion with the angle of pull between 20 and 30°.

The decision in favor of surgical intervention is based on objective neurologic deficit that does not respond to or benefit from conservative treatment; poses a functional loss; and is confirmed as to etiology by CT scan, MRI, or myelogram. The choice of technique is then the prerogative of the surgeon.

Diskectomy, nuclectomy, anterior or posterior approach, with or without fusion, anterior interbody or posterior laminar fusion—choice of technique depends on the surgeon's opinion, expertise, competence, and experience. The prognosis is also the surgeon's responsibility as to morbidity/complications from surgery, the duration of convalescence, the prognosis for possible recovery or residual loss and the needed postoperative treatment: all reside with the surgeon.

Conservative Nonsurgical Treatment of the Herniated Cervical Disk

The treatment of the patient with a confirmed herniated cervical disk and neurologic deficit is essentially that of the patient with any cervical diskogenic painful syndrome.

The aspects of treatment can be itemized as follows:

1. Rest of the part
2. Modalities to the cervical spine
3. Medications for the symptoms
4. Immobilization
5. Mobilization
   a. Manipulation
   b. Exercise
6. Traction

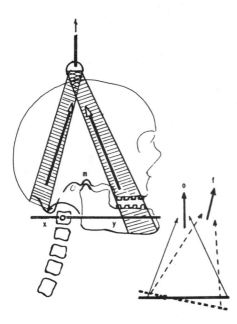

Figure 7–24. Angle of traction on head halter. The head halter superimposed upon the skull depicts the short lever arm and small point of attachment at the base of the skull, x, and the longer lever arm under the chin at y. If traction is from direction o, the longer arm would tend to extend the neck; but by advancing the traction above and ahead of the head, the direction of pull tends to cause neck flexion. It is evident that the pressure from traction arm y is concentrated on the teeth and at the temporomandibular joint, m.

7. "Neck school"
   a.   Posture
   b   ADL
8. Psychologic intervention
   a.   Tension/anxiety
   b.   Depression
   c.   Compensation neurosis

Rest. The *modality* of rest is more applicable to the acute injury, but it needs clarification when applied to the resultant disk herniation. Minimizing any activity that may aggravate the symptoms of neck or arm pain is desirable. Minimizing excessive driving, avoiding stressful situations, minimizing work at the computer, and so forth can be construed as *rest*. Bed rest or reclining in a comfortable position for brief periods, thus relieving the stress of gravity on the neck, also may be of value.

Modalities. Application of ice or heat, electrical stimulation, ultrasound, pressure point, massage, and acupressure tend to give subjective relief but are, per se, not specifically therapeutic. Therefore none should be employed as a sole therapeutic modality at the expense of the patient's time, effort, travel, or financial burden. The main value of these modalities is as an accompaniment to exercise. Heat and ice can be applied easily and frequently as a home activity. Both decrease the protective muscular spasm and the limitation of neck motion, but they have minimal effect on the more deeply situated nerve roots in the foramina or on the intervertebral disk.

Medication. There are numerous medications that have been employed in the treatment of the herniated cervical disk. Many have palliative benefit in that they help relieve pain and apprehension in the patient.

Oral steroids have been claimed to be specific in relieving inflammation of the disk and of the nerve roots, the latter of which are also undergoing swelling and fibrous reaction (Frykholm). It is postulated that steroids act on the nerve roots in a manner that can obviate ultimate surgery. Steroids have never been shown to decrease the irritating reaction of the entrapped nerve root or to have a direct specific effect on the disk matrix proteoglycans or annulus fibers (Ghosh). Steroids may have an antiphlogistic effect and may decrease the painful reaction of the patient who is undergoing natural recovery or healing.

The use of epidural steroids, recently advocated by Warfield and associates, has yet to be controlled or randomized, and only a small number of patients have been treated with them. It has been shown that its use decreases the symptoms but does not improve the strength of the involved myotome nor necessarily decrease the objective hypalgesia. Epidural steroids must, therefore, still be considered palliative and experimental. Administration technique is difficult and not mastered by many at this date.

Muscle relaxants also have been attributed a role in relieving the painful effect of the resultant protective muscle *spasm* incurred by the irritated nerve root. No scientific basis has been proven that any currently known drug is truly a muscle *relaxant*. The effect of so-called muscle relaxants is probably that of an anxiety/apprehension depressant, and in that capacity these medications are of value in relieving pain and protective *spasm*. (The term *spasm* is italicized due to the fact that where there has been clinically diagnosed "spasm" no evidence of extrafusal fiber contraction has ever been documented on EMG examination.)

Because chronic sustained muscle contraction (increased tone) enhances the undesirable effect on the disk herniation, a decrease in this unwanted muscle tension can be considered of value. External muscular contraction, especially when sustained, is accepted as a contributing factor in the increase of disk pressure.

Immobilization. A collar (Fig. 7–21) or a cervical brace (Fig. 7–22) that immobilizes the neck in a physiologic position has been found to be of great value. The correct posture intended is placing and maintaining the head directly over the center of gravity, thus minimizing significant flexion or extension and the amount of lateral flexion and rotation. This physiologic posture decreases the cervical lordosis and thus maintains adequate opening of the foramina, decreases the amount of added pressure upon the nerve root, and minimizes the irregular pressure upon the disk.

By supporting the head in a minimal lordosis and directly above the center of gravity, a *brace* also decreases the need for external muscles to splint the neck and to support the head.

The judicious use of a brace, support, or collar is of value, but a word of

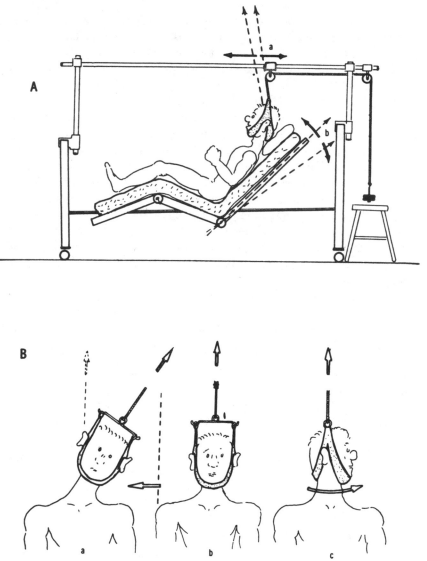

Figure 7–25. Bed cervical traction, hospital type. (*A*) The patient should be seated in a slightly flexed position with hips and knees flexed and low back relaxed. The traction should come from above and ahead of the trunk. Pulley, a, may be moved ahead or behind to alter direction of traction. The neck, however, should always be flexed. The line of pull may be altered by changing inclination of the bed, b. A stool should be under the weights so that the distance is very short in case of a sudden drop or fall. The stool is also convenient for the periods during which the traction is released. A monkey bar may be hung from the overhead bar for the patient's convenience. (*B*) The manner of direct traction with head straight ahead, b, and with head rotated, c. By laterally shifting the body, a, the traction causes lateral stretch as well as direct traction.

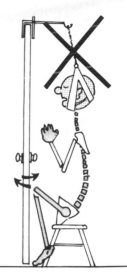

Figure 7–26. Ineffective home door cervical traction. The patient is too close to the door to receive correct neck flexion angle. The door freely opens and closes, not permitting constant traction. The patient cannot extend the legs or assume a comfortable position. This type of home traction is not recommended.

caution is mandatory. Prolonged use of a neck brace without all other approaches of treatment, such as exercise and posture and ADL training, may be detrimental. The patient must be monitored constantly as to the status of the nerve deficit. If there is improvement—that is, diminution of nerve deficit—the patient should be "weaned" from the collar gradually to encourage him or her to use more physiologic methods such as exercise. If there is continuation or progression of nerve deficit, the use of the collar is obviously inappropriate treatment, and other methods of treatment must be considered.

Mobilization. This category can be divided into *mobilization* and *manipulation*. *Mobilization* concerns external force applied to increase the range of motion but with no *thrust* at the end of the range to gain the added range. Both mobilization and manipulation aim to gain greater mobility or to overcome immobility.

"Manipulation therapy is concerned with relief of symptoms through the restoration of normal motion. Normal range of motion (ROM) is not synonymous with normal motion . . . which implies that controls of motion also must be normal" (Farfan). Joint range of motion is inhibited (restricted) from ligamentous restriction, capsular limitation, cartilaginous changes of the articular surfaces (facets), or muscular limitation.

The intervertebral disk is not a direct mechanical factor in this limitation by virtue of annular protrusion, tear, or nuclear herniation. A herniated intervertebral disk, whether it is internal nuclear or external annular, has not been considered *mechanically* to immobilize a functional unit. A herniated disk prob-

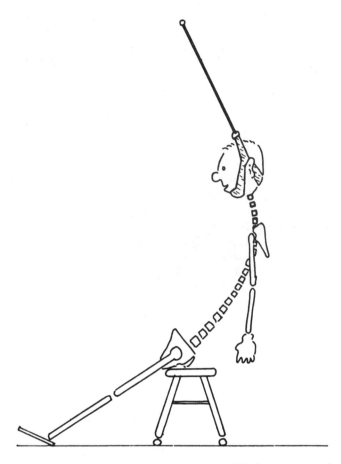

Figure 7–27. Overhead cervical traction for home use. With the rope securely fastened overhead and slightly in front of the seated patient, the traction is applied on the flexed neck. The patient should be seated in a fully relaxed position with low back flexed, legs extended, and arms dangling at his side. This position attains maximum relaxation.

ably immobilizes motion by concomitant muscular spasm. To manipulate a cervical vertebral functional unit to return (reduce) the nucleus to within the annular confines of the disk is an untenable concept. Magnetic resonance imaging or CT scanning after a manipulation has never revealed reduction of disk herniation.

The disk has no free range of motion (Farfan), and force is needed to achieve motion of the disk. The disk has a stiffness because of its intrinsic hydrodynamic pressure and from the tension of the annular sheets in their oblique radiation. Physiologic rotation of 5° has been postulated. Further rotation (more

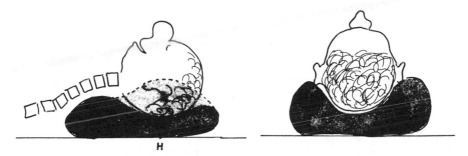

H

Figure 7–28. Cervical pillow. There are numerous commercial brands and designs, but most are shaped to fill in the cervical lordosis to a degree yet support the head (H) at the occiput to maintain slight neck flexion. The pillow also cradles the head on each side to prevent lateral flexion and rotation.

than 5°) is therefore unphysiologic and interrupts the normal stiffness of the disk.

Forceful manipulation to increase rotary range of motion, therefore, can only possibly incur further damage to a disk the annulus of which has sustained tearing with internal extrusion of the nucleus. That manipulation changes the relationship of the annular bulge against the taut nerve root has never been confirmed and has been postulated only by clinical relief of radiculitis.

The facets of the functional unit may be freed (regain range of motion) from manipulation. How and if this occurs is also speculation, varying from (1) freeing an entrapped synovial fold, (2) unlocking a disk within the facet joint (which has been anatomically described but denied by many anatomists), or (3) breakup of the reflex muscular spasm via acute Golgi and spindle system stimulation. Currently it can be stated that whatever clinical benefit can be derived from manipulation has no confirmed physiologic basis.

Mobilization does benefit the impaired functional unit by elongating the ligamentous, capsular, and muscle fascia restraints, but the effect upon the bulging annulus or nucleus with entrapment of the nerve root and its dura is unproven. In the recovering annulus bulge with nerve root entrapment mobilization restores normal physiologic motion of the spine and assists in preventing relapses or recurrences.

Traction. Traction has been employed since antiquity for the treatment of cervical disease. The concept has been based on *distraction* of the affected functional units. This distracting force allegedly (1) decreases the cervical lordosis, (2) opens the intervertebral foramina, (3) overcomes the protective muscular spasm of the cervical musculature, (4) nullifies the effects of gravity, and (5) therefore untraps the nerve root compression.

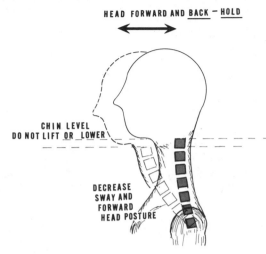

HEAD FORWARD AND <u>BACK</u> — <u>HOLD</u>

CHIN LEVEL
DO NOT LIFT <u>OR LOWER</u>

DECREASE
SWAY AND
FORWARD
HEAD POSTURE

Figure 7–29. Exercise to decrease lordosis and forward head posture.

NECK STRENGTHENING 1

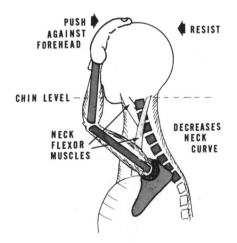

PUSH
AGAINST
FOREHEAD

RESIST

CHIN LEVEL —

NECK
FLEXOR
MUSCLES

DECREASES
NECK
CURVE

Figure 7–30. Neck strengthening 1.

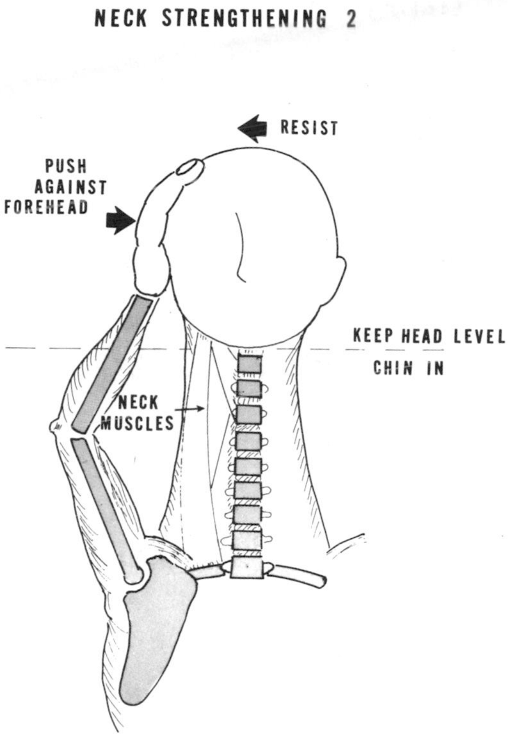

NECK STRENGTHENING 2

Figure 7–31. Neck strengthening 2.

Any or all of these benefits may be operational, and a period of traction is justified when a diagnosis of cervical disk herniation with radiculitis has been made. There is also a better expectation from traction if the head traction test (see Fig. 7–12) described earlier decreases or eliminates the radicular symptoms.

Traction can be applied manually or mechanically.

In the manual method the therapist applies traction to the neck by holding the patient's head between two hands and pulling steadily at an angle of approximately 20° flexion. The duration and the force applied is determined by the response of the patient and the ability of the therapist. Usually the angulation, duration, and force of this technique is accepted by the patient, who can express how it feels and how it helps the symptoms. The undesirable aspect of this method is that it requires a therapist who can apply traction for only a limited time with variable force and at variable frequencies. This is why mechanical traction, which can be applied by the patient with frequency, duration, and force

LIFTING

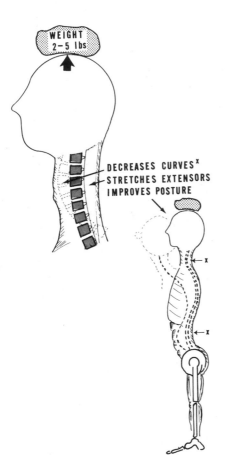

Figure 7–32. Posture exercise: Distraction.

is usually advocated. Manual traction does, however, indicate whether the patient will tolerate or benefit from traction and at what angle, duration, and force.

Of the available mechanical methods of applying cervical traction, the horizontal method appears to be the most effective and best tolerated. Because the force of traction is applied by the patient, the maximum traction accepted will be exerted (Fig. 7–23).

The angulation considered most effective is usually 20° of neck flexion (Fig. 7–24) applied for 20 minutes 3–6 times daily. Concurrent with traction, the application of a hot moist pack around the neck helps relax the muscles and permits the patient to tolerate the traction.

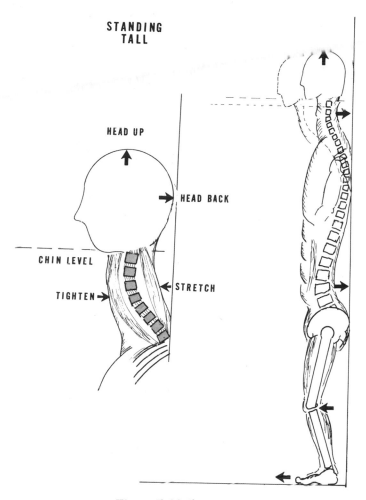

STANDING TALL

HEAD UP

HEAD BACK

CHIN LEVEL

STRETCH

TIGHTEN

Figure 7–33. Posture exercise.

Should the radicular symptoms be severe and reasonably acute, home or hospital bed traction is very effective (Fig. 7–25). In addition to direct overhead traction, a slight side traction will open the foramina on the side away from which the traction is applied. Some rotation of the head during traction also affords benefit.

Home cervical traction using an over-the-door traction setup (Fig. 7–26) has, in my opinion, been ineffectual and least easily utilized. A better method of home traction is shown in Figure 7–27.

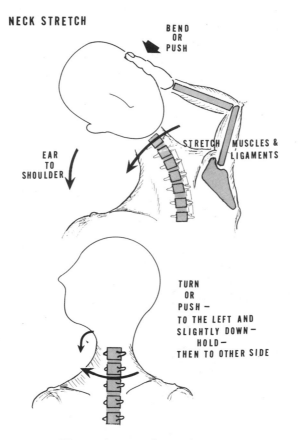

NECK STRETCH

BEND
OR
PUSH

EAR
TO
SHOULDER

STRETCH MUSCLES &
LIGAMENTS

TURN
OR
PUSH —
TO THE LEFT AND
SLIGHTLY DOWN —
HOLD —
THEN TO OTHER SIDE

Figure 7–34. Neck stretch exercise.

Sleeping position can also be maintained to afford relief by the use of a cervical pillow (Fig. 7–28). There are numerous types on the market that can be used if found to be comfortable. Comfort is the criterion for a specific type of pillow.

Exercises. The value of exercises in the presence of clinically diagnosed herniated cervical disk is primarily to (1) decrease cervical lordosis and the forward-head posture (Fig. 7–29), (2) strengthen the short neck flexors (Fig. 7–30), (3) improve posture for ADL (Figs. 7–31 to 7–33).

Flexibility (Fig. 7–34) is also gained from exercise, as well as strength to maintain proper posture.

Neck School. Just as the value of *the back school* has been proven effective in the treatment of low back pain to decrease pain, impairment, and to prevent recurrence, so can a *neck school* accomplish the same purpose.

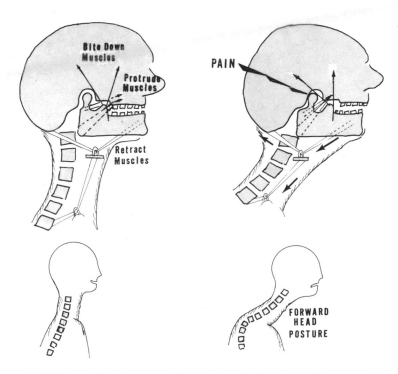

Figure 7–35. Forward-head posture. With the head held ahead of the center of gravity, there is neck strain and other postural defects. Good posture aligns the entire body along the center of gravity.

The "curriculum" of the school is essentially the following:

1. Instructions in the basics of neck anatomy
2. Instructions on proper exercise and its value
3. Instructions in proper posture (Figs. 7–35 to 7–37)
4. Instructions in the application of proper body mechanics in every aspect of ADL—at home, at work, in the car, and so forth (Figs. 7–38 to 7–40)
5. Instruction in how the emotions affect the posture and impair the control of muscles, leading to damage of the tissues of the cervical spine.

Psychologic Intervention. Upon determining that the afflicted patient has significant psychologic problems that may be related to the cervical component, psychologic intervention must be initiated. Having instructed and oriented the patient in the relationship between tension, anxiety, depression, anger, impatience, and so forth, to the muscles, ligaments, and disks of the cervical

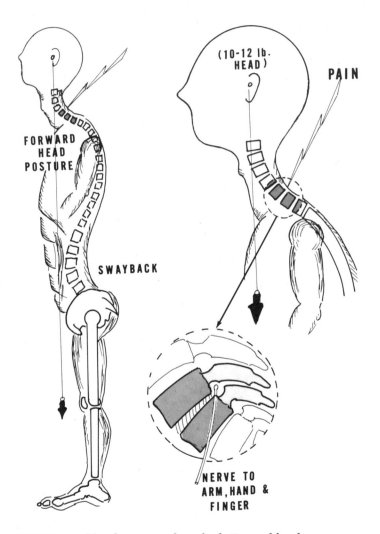

Figure 7–36. Forward-head posture and swayback. Forward-head posture causes an increase in the cervical lordosis and closes the foramina, entrapping the nerve roots.

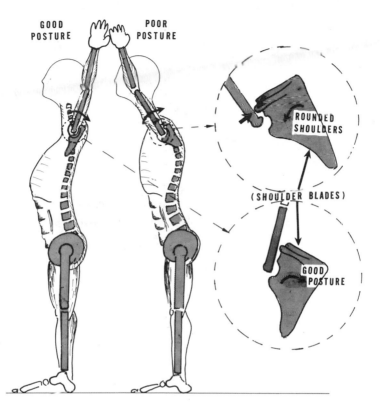

Figure 7–37. Good posture, poor posture. Poor posture causes "round shoulders" with downward rotation of the scapula, entrapping the rotator cuffs of the gleno humeral joints.

spine, the psychologic problem must be discussed in a language understandable to the patient. There must not be any implication of accusation—"It's all in your head," "Your problems are tension," "You are nervous," and so forth. An explanation that is understood by the patient to be sympathetic results in assurance and assists in directing him or her toward accepting and undertaking psychologic assistance.

Muscular tension, albeit of emotional origin, has an adverse effect on the tissues of the cervical spine, especially the muscles and the disks. Biofeedback, self-hypnosis, and psychologic guidance such as stress management are effective.

Treatment of depression as it relates to any painful part of the musculoskeletal system or to chronic pain needs no amplification here. In addition to medications and psychotherapy, treatment of depression must include addressing physical postural components of depression.

AVOID

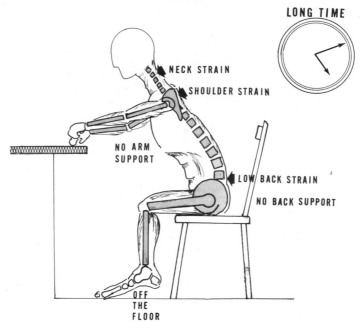

Figure 7–38. Sitting posture to avoid

AVOID

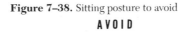

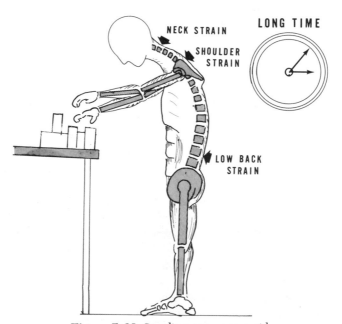

Figure 7–39. Standing posture to avoid.

IDEAL SITTING

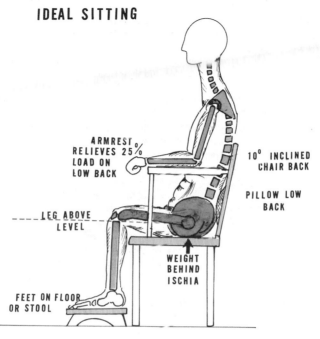

Figure 7–40. Ideal sitting posture: All aspects of proper sitting posture are depicted here.

Chronic pain is persistence of the symptoms of the acute pain, impairment, and disability for more than 6 weeks after most of the acute manifestations have subsided. This condition merits a full discussion, but it can be briefly stated that many cases of chronic pain are the result of inadequate acute treatment. Early recognition of the patient with a deep-seated emotional problem, as well as of the mechanical aspect of cervical diskogenic disease, is the first step in prevention of chronic pain.

The acronym SAD is used in the treatment of the cervical diskogenic syndrome. The S stands for somatic symptoms. The A represents anxiety, apprehension, and anger. The D stands for drugs, dependency, depression, discouragement, and disuse disability. All must be addressed and avoided to prevent chronicity.

BIBLIOGRAPHY

Adams, CBT and Logue, V: Studies in cervical spondylotic myelopathy. I. Movement of the cervical roots, dura and cord, and their relation to the course of the extradural roots. Brain 94:557, 1971.

Benini, A: Clinical Features of Cervical Root Compression C5-C8 and Their Variations. Neuro-Orthopedics 4, 74, 1987.

Brieg, A: Biomechanics of the Central Nervous System. Almquist and Wiksell, Stockholm, 1960.

Cailliet, R: Soft Tissue Pain and Disability, ed 2. FA Davis, Philadelphia, 1988.

Cailliet, R: Low Back Pain Syndrome, ed 4. FA Davis, Philadelphia, 1988.

Cailliet, R and Gross, L: The Rejuvenation Strategy. Doubleday & Co, New York, 1987.

Cloward, RB: Lesions of the Intervertebral Disk and their treatment by interbody fusion method. Clin Orthop 27:51, 1963.

Cloward, RB: Cervical diskography: A contribution to the etiology and mechanism of neck shoulder and arm pain. Ann Surg 150:1052, 1959.

Denslow, JS, Korr, IM, and Krems, AD: Quantitative studies of chronic fascilitation in human mononeuron pools. Am J Physiol 150:229, 1947.

Elliott, FA and Kremer, M: Brachial pain from herniation of cervical intervertebral disk. Lancet 1:4, 1944.

Farfan, HF: The scientific basis of manipulative procedures. Clin Rheum Dis 6(1)159, 1980.

Frykholm, R: Deformities of dural pouches and structures of dural sheaths in cervical region producing nerve root compression: Contribution to etiology and operative treatment of brachial neuralgia. J Neurosurg 4:403, 1947.

Frykholm, R: Cervical nerve root compression resulting from disc degeneration and root sleeve fibrosis: A clinical investigation. Acta Chir Scand (Suppl) 160, 1951.

Ghosh, P: Influence of drugs, hormones and other agents on the metabolism of the disc and sequelae of its degeneration. In Ghosh P(ed): The Biology of the Intervertebral Disc, vol 11. CRC Press, Boca Raton, FL, 1988.

Gordon, EE: Natural history of the intervertebral disc. Arch Phys Med Rehab 42:750, 1961.

Howe, F, Loeser, JD, and Calvin, WJ: Mechanosensitivity of dorsal root ganglia and chronically injured axons: A physiological basis for radicular pain of nerve root compression. 2nd World Congress of Pain, Montreal, Pain (abstr) 1:217, 1978.

Jackson, R: The Cervical Syndrome, ed 2. Charles C Thomas, Springfield, IL, 1958.

Khan, MRH, McInnes, A, and Hughes, SPF: Electrophysiological studies in cervical spondylosis. Journal of Spinal Disorders 2(3):163, 1989.

Michelsen, JJ and Mixter, WJ: Pain and disability of shoulder girdle and arm due to herniation of the nucleus pulposus of cervical intervertebral disks. N Engl J Med 231:279, 1944.

Reed, JD: Effects of flexion-extension movements of the head and spine upon the spinal cord and nerve roots. J Neurol Neurosurg Psychiatry 23:214, 1960.

Roofe, RP: Innervation of annulus fibrosus and posterior longitudinal ligaments, fourth and fifth lumbar level. Arch Neurol Psychiat 44:100–103, 1940.

Shea, AP, Wood, WW, and Werder, DH: Electromyography in the diagnosis of nerve root compression syndrome. Arch Neurol Psychiatry 69:93, 1950.

Turner, EL and Oppenheimer, A: A common lesion of the cervical spine responsible for segmental neuritis. Ann Intern Med 10:427, 1936.

Vernon-Roberts, B: Disc pathology and disease states. In Ghosh, P (ed): The Biology of the Intervertebral Disc, vol 11. CRC Press, Boca Raton, FL, 1988.

Viikari-Juntura, E, Porras, M, and Laasonen, EM: Validity of Clinical Tests in the Diagnosis of Root Compression in Cervical Disc Disease. Spine 14 (3):23, 1989.

Warfield, CA, et al: Epidural steroid injection as a treatment for cervical radiculitis. Clin J Pain 4:201, 1988.

Wedell, G, Feinstein, B, and Prattle, A: The clinical application of electromyography. Lancet 1:236, 1945.

CHAPTER 8

Spondylosis: Degenerative Disk Disease

Spondylosis is a term for a condition of pathologic change in the spinal column. The term has several synonyms, such as *degenerative disk disease, degenerative spondylosis, osteophytosis,* and *spondylitis deformans.* It is a vertebral ankylosis (immobility of a joint).

Clinically, cervical spondylosis undoubtedly plays a greater role in producing neck pain and nerve root radiculopathy than does the *ruptured disk* discussed in the preceding chapter. This statement, however, may be redundant inasmuch as some disk bulging, a variant of disk herniation, with nerve root compression or encroachment upon the posterior longitudinal ligament, is a frequent sequela of degenerative disk disease.

There currently is a paucity of precise laboratory or clinical studies on the etiology, causation, development, evolution, and clinical manifestation of spondylosis despite the fact that it is frequently diagnosed radiologically (Vernon-Roberts and Pirie).

Schmorl and Junghanns' report upon findings in autopsies of 4253 spines found evidence of spondylosis in 60 percent of women and 80 percent of men by the age of 49 years. He found 95 percent incidence in both sexes at age 70 years. Significant structural changes in the disk have been reported in most studies of pathologic disks in patients past the age of 30 to 35 years.

Spondylosis is a term applied to changes noted in the spine of radiologically significant (1) narrowing of the disk height, (2) presence of osteophytes arising from the disk margins, and (3) osteoarthritic changes in the posterior zygapophyseal joints.

The diagnosis of spondylosis is made by radiologic changes noted in routine examination of symptomatic patients, and the "condition" is considered to be the cause of symptoms of neck pain, neck motion limitation, and/or referred arm/hand/finger pain.

More recently the use of MRI has shed light on earlier changes within the disk than those revealed in x-ray examinations. It is hoped that better evaluation and chronologic studies of pathology will emerge from these and related studies.

There remains controversy as to whether spondylotic changes in the spine must be regarded as the inevitable change of aging or whether these degenerative changes are the result of some unidentified series of events, such as trauma, faulty posture, anxiety, or genetic weakness.

The specific mechanism for the formation of osteophytes remains controversial. What is not controversial is that the presence of osteophytes is mechanically responsible for encroachment upon neural tissues—nerve root and/or spinal cord—with resultant neurologic symptoms.

Disk nutrition has been well-studied (Maroudas), and it is accepted that the vascular supply to the intervertebral disk is obliterated by calcification of the vertebral endplates at puberty. Disk nutrition is the response considered to occur by diffusion from variable solute concentrations which are transported into the disk via (1) blood vessels surrounding the disk and (2) blood vessels in the subchondral layers of the endplates.

By variations of alternating compressive forces, *imbibition* has been postulated to be as important in nutrition of the disk as it is in cartilage, but some questions regarding this mechanism in disk nutrition are arising. Studies (Maroudas) have indicated that hydraulic permeability of the disk matrix is very low, whereas solute diffusivity is very high. This would indicate greater infusion of nutritive solutes via diffusion than by imbibition. The method by which the disk receives its nutrition is not yet confirmed.

Degeneration of the disk is considered to begin within the annulus as slight tears of the annular fibers. These tears apparently begin in the vicinity of the nucleus, ascend-descend toward the endplates, then migrate outward. Initially the nuclear material remains encapsulated within the inner annular fibers, but the nucleus undergoes gradual changes, becoming more dense and undergoing changes in its inner collagen fibers.

The nucleus gradually emerges through the fissures within the annulus. The outer annular fibers remain essentially intact but separate and allow invasion between the layers. Due to the weakening of the inner annulus there is a change in the gradient pressure, and the disk annulus *bulges* (Fig. 8–1).

As the disk degenerates, it also dehydrates. The intradiskal pressure decreases, but the disk does not significantly narrow. The inner pressure gradient balances the forces of gravity and the external muscular tonus.

OSTEOPHYTOSIS

Osteophytosis, the formation of osteophytes, remains controversial as to the exact mechanism of formation. Collins postulated that these osteophytes

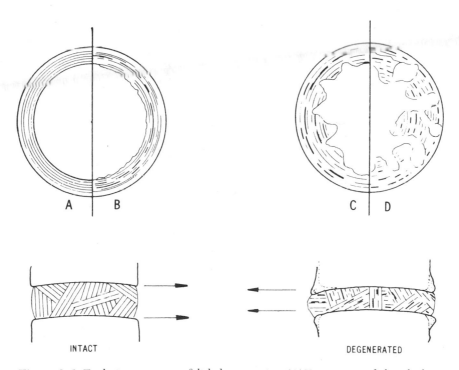

Figure 8–1. Evolutionary stages of disk degeneration. *(A)* Young, intact disk with elastic annular fibers and a well-hydrated nucleus. *(B)* Early stages of degeneration reveal fibrillation of the annulus, some fragmentation, and beginning dehydration of the annulus. *(C)* Moderate stage shows a furtherance of *B* with early invasion of the annulus by fragments of the nucleus. *(D)* Advanced stage of degeneration is that of marked nuclear dehydration and fragmentation with invasion of the shredded annulus, permitting nuclear fragments to reach the periphery of the disk, where only the ligamentous structures remain.

form as the result of internal disk pressure dissecting the longitudinal ligaments away from the vertebral periosteum (Fig. 8–2). The internal pressure allowed the nuclear material to fill in between the vertebral body and the longitudinal ligament. A refutation of this concept has been raised (Vernon-Roberts), pointing out that although the anterior longitudinal ligament, unlike the posterior longitudinal ligament, is not contiguous or part of the outer annulus, anterior osteophytes occur as often as posterior osteophytes.

Recent studies do not support the theory of longitudinal ligament dissection with subsequent invasion of nuclear material and its ossification, because microscopically there is no new subperiosteal bone formation. Studies by Vernon-Roberts and Pirie indicate endochondral ossification within the annulus where the annular fibers attach to the cartilage of the endplates. Regardless of

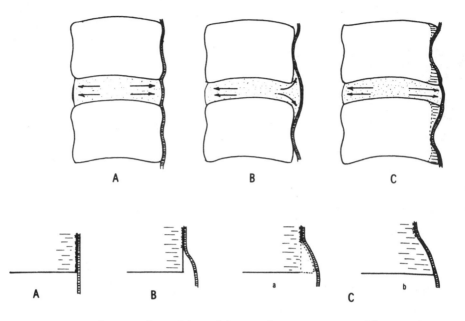

Figure 8–2. Mechanism of spondylosis. (A) Normal anterior portion of functional unit with an intact disk, normal interspace, and a taut posterior longitudinal ligament that is totally adherent to the vertebral body periosteum. (B) Disk degeneration permits approximation of the two vertebrae, causing a slack in the posterior longitudinal ligament. The intradiskal pressure dissects the ligament away from the periosteum, and disk material intervenes. (C) Extruded disk material becomes fibrous (a), then calcifies into a *spur* (b).

the evolution of formation, the osteophytes develop as sequela to disk degeneration.

Because of the presence of the uncovertebral joints of von Luschka, osteophytosis (Fig. 8–3) is of greater incidence in the cervical spine than in the lumbar spine, where these joints do not exist. Because the uncovertebral joints are *pseudojoints*—essentially exostoses—they have no cartilage intervening, and, being approximating articulating osteoarthroses, they enlarge and deform from repeated friction, compression, and abrasion.

Anteriorly the vertebral bodies approximate and the vertebral osteophytes form. Posteriorly the zygapophyseal joints also approximate as the anterior portion narrows. These joints undergo asymmetrical motion and compression (Fig. 8–4) due to instability of the functional unit. The cartilage of the zygapophyseal joints undergoes degenerative changes which can be considered typical degenerative articular changes, termed *osteoarthritis* (Fig. 8–5).

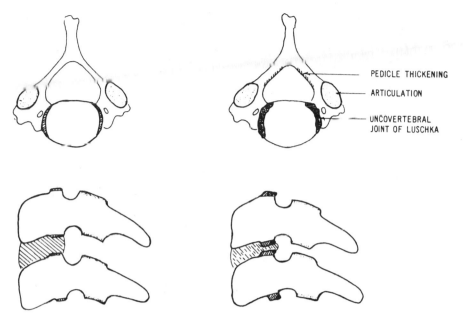

PEDICLE THICKENING

ARTICULATION

UNCOVERTEBRAL
JOINT OF LUSCHKA

Figure 8–3. Disk degeneration with formation of *spondylosis*. *(Left)* Normal relationship of the vertebral bodies separated by an intact disk, normal uncovertebral joints of von Luschka, and normal posterior articulations (facets). *(Right)* Changes resulting from disk degeneration. The vertebral bodies approximate; the uncovertebral joints thicken, roughen, and distort; the foramina deform; and the facets thicken and also deform. These drawings do not show the additional soft tissue changes, such as thickening of the longitudinal ligaments and thickening and curling of the ligamentum flavum. The facet capsules also thicken. All these soft tissue changes plus the boney changes shown narrow the intervertebral foramina and the interspinal canal.

SYMPTOMATOLOGY OF CERVICAL SPONDYLOSIS

The end result of these degenerative changes in the cervical spine is that the following sequelae may occur.

The narrowed disk spaces limit normal range of motion of the anterior aspect of the functional unit. The longitudinal ligaments undergo thickening and loss of elongation (plasticity). Clinically the neck undergoes limited range of motion with or without pain and discomfort. The patient becomes aware of an inability to move the head and neck as before. Unless this limitation interferes with ADL no complaint is rendered, and only upon examination is the loss noted. Flexion and rotation surprisingly remain satisfactory, inasmuch as 30 to 40° of flexion-extension and 75 to 90° of rotation occur at the occipital cervical level (occiput-atlas-axis), where similar degenerative changes do not occur because

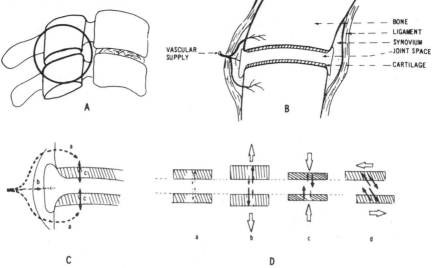

Figure 8–4. Normal nutrition and lubrication of posterior articulation (facet). *(A)* The posterior articulation, the zygapophyseal joint. This cervical joint is a diarthroidial joint containing a capsule, synovium, joint space containing fluid, and two articular cartilages; it is supplied by its unique vascular bed. *(B, C)* Diffusion cycle to cartilage nutrition. The arterial supply separates into a capillary bed to bone (a), and a capillary bed to the synovium (b). Cartilage nutrition is by diffusion through the cartilage (c) from both capillary beds by spongelike compression and expansion of the cartilage. *(D)* Mechanism of cartilage nutrition. (a) No imbibition with joint at rest. (b) Inflow from relaxation or joint extension. (c) Squeezing out of synovial fluid by cartilage compression. (d) Creation of lubrication layer between surfaces by motion between two incongruent surfaces.

of the anatomic differences from the lower cervical vertebrae (see Chapter 1).

If trauma is superimposed—such as an external mechanical trauma, acute recurrent tension-anxiety, or faulty postural changes—inflammation results within the nociceptive tissues of the vertebrae, resulting in pain and limitation of range of motion. These nociceptive sites are the facet capsules, cervical ligaments and muscles, and the neural contents of the foramina.

The symptoms of pain (discussed earlier) occur, and now the added x-ray finding of *degenerative arthritis* is reported. There is a tendency to impute this arthritis as the cause of pain, whereas it is the trauma and the resultant inflamed nociceptive tissue sites within a degenerated spine that cause pain.

The cervical spondylosis also causes changes in the width and depth of the intervertebral foramina (Fig. 8–6). As the foramina narrow, the space permitted the nerve roots with their dural sheaths is restricted. This exposes the nerve roots to further injury if any superimposed trauma occurs, such as external trauma, anxiety-tension, or faulty posture (Figs. 8–7, 8–8).

The predominant sites of osteophyte formation in the entire spine are at

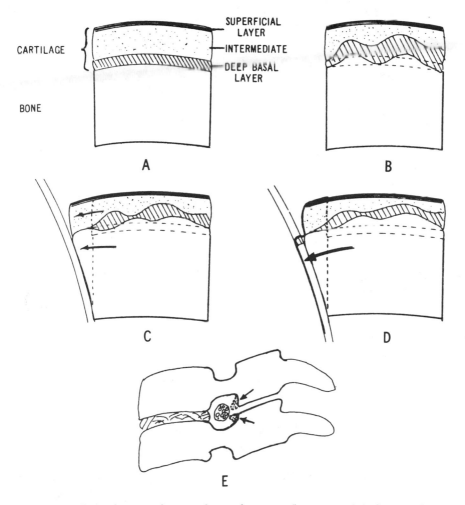

Figure 8–5. Mechanism of osteoarthritic changes in facet joints. (A) The articular cartilage consists of three layers: (1) superficial tangential layer of collagen fibers, (2) an intermediate spongy, shock-absorbing layer, and (3) a deep, calcified, basal layer that is firmly bound to the subchondral bone. (B) Wear and tear causes new bone formation of the subchondral plate and thickening of the calcified basal layer with lengthening of the bone. (C) Peripheral lateral growth widens the end of the bone. (D) Finally, the ligaments ossify. (E) Encroachment into the intervertebral foramen from osteoarthritis.

the summits of concavity, the points furthest from the center of gravity. As shown in Figure 8–7, these sites are at C-4 to C-5 and C-5 to C-6. Their presence at these sites, incidentally, also lends credence to the theory that osteophytes occur at the sites of mechanical irritation and compression

Neurologic radiculopathy can thus occur from cervical spondylosis. Ac-

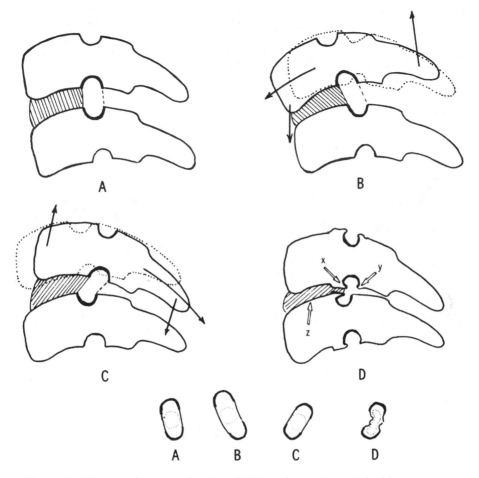

Figure 8–6. Foraminal opening variations. (A)Normal open intervertebral foramen with the neck in a neutral, slightly flexed position and not rotated or laterally tilted to either side. (B) Flexion, which occurs below C-3, by forward gliding of the upper upon the lower vertebra, maintains full opening. (C) Extension by backward gliding of the upper upon the lower vertebra normally narrows the foraminal aperture. (D) Degenerated disk and osteophyte formation from the joints of von Luschka (not even considering the soft tissue components). Comparison with normal (A) shows the marked encroachment upon the foraminal space.

cepting that the normal foramina close upon cervical extension and on the side toward which the neck turns explains why nerve root symptoms can be aggravated upon examination by initiating these motions. The presence of osteophytes and narrowing of intervertebral foramina explains the susceptibility of nerve root entrapment. Motion—extension and/or rotation—intensifies the

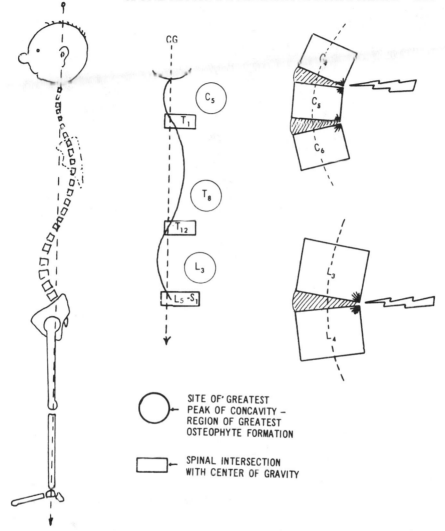

Figure 8–7. Sites of greatest osteophyte formation. The lateral view of the static erect spine (posture) demonstrates the sites of transection of the spine with the plumb line of gravity (external ear meatus, odontoid process, T-11, T-12, and sacral promontory). The greatest points of pressure, thus the sites of osteophyte formation, are at the points of greatest concavity, furthest from the plumb line (C-5, T-8, L-3).

pressure of the osteophyte on the nerve root.

Faulty posture clearly may intensify the propensity of nerve root entrapment. Prolonged faulty posture may not, however, cause nerve root symptoms, because the nerve roots adapt to gradual prolonged compression (Brain).

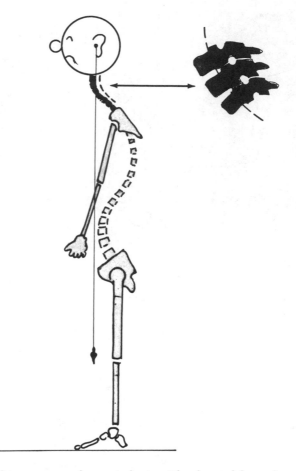

Figure 8–8. Effect of posture upon the cervical spine. The slumped forward posture causes the head to be held ahead of the center of gravity. The cervical spine must assume a greater lordosis to balance and thus closes the intervertebral foramina and places more pressure upon the zygapophyseal (facet) joints.

CERVICAL RADICULOPATHY
FROM SPONDYLOSIS

There have been studies to correlate the extent of nerve root impairment with the degree of degenerative diskogenic disease, but the results remain unclear. The reason for neuropathy also has undergone study, but there has been no conclusion regarding the exact pathomechanics.

There is no doubt that the degree of disk degeneration directly influences the degree of nerve root entrapment and nerve root pathology. There also remains sufficient residual intradiskal pressure within the nucleus to exert peripheral pressure. This pressure may force disk matrix and annulus against the longitudinal ligament, and the intervertebral foramen against the nerve root. Disk herniation may coexist with disk and zygapophyseal degenerative changes and cause symptoms. This possibility justifies doing confirmatory radiologic studies if neuropathy is objectively present.

This protruding disk material is often termed a *soft disk herniation*. Ultimately the protrusion acquires a preponderence of fibrous tissue, forming what is known as a *hard disk*. Calcification of the protruding fibrous disk material becomes a *spur*, or osteophyte.

Degenerative changes occur in asymptomatic people and in patients with normal x-ray findings. The presence of osteophytes invading the intervertebral foramina on radiologic studies does not necessarily result in nerve root irritation (Tapiovaara and Heinevaara). Also, degenerative changes within the zygapophyseal joints can occur without significant intervertebral disk degeneration, which implies that there are many unrecognized mechanical or chemical factors that can alter otherwise normal functional unit structures (Horwitz; Holt and Yates).

Trauma superimposed upon a structurally sound and asymptomatic cervical spine may result in symptoms. A degenerated spine is obviously less resilient to trauma than a normal spine.

It is of clinical interest that the nerve root lesions are usually limited to the posterior nerve root, the nerve root ganglion, or the junction of the root and the ganglion. Clinically, sensory manifestations of trauma or injury rather than motor symptoms are noted by patients. Dermatomal loss of sensation, termed *numbness* or *tingling*, is a frequent claim by patients. Pain, numbness, or discomfort may be localized by the patient as being in the interscapular area (C_5 to C_6), the upper extremity (C_5 to C_6), the thumb (C_6), or the ring and little fingers (C_7 to C_8).

The reason for this sensory involvement rather than motor deficit is that the nerve root normally divides into two distinct roots (in 50 percent of cases) at the neural foraminal level.

The sensory root lies in proximity to the posterior zygapophyseal joints, and, hence, encroachment upon this posterior (sensory) root leads to sensory symptomatology rather than motor deficit (Fig. 8 9). This is also why electromyography (EMG) test results may be negative (Waylonis), inasmuch as the motor roots are usually spared. Sensory conduction times, which test only the peripheral nerve and not the roots, are also negative in symptomatic patients.

The nerve roots usually involved are in the mid cervical and lower cervical regions because the nerve roots are more vulnerable to trauma in these regions. In cervical motion it is accepted that the nerve roots are usually displaced backward and laterally. This movement of the nerve roots may cause the nerve roots to be stretched or angulated over the boney prominences that encroach into the

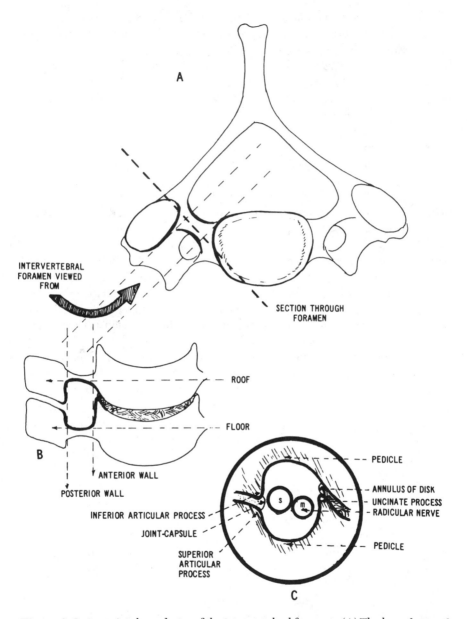

Figure 8–9. Anatomic boundaries of the intervertebral foramen. *(A)* The boundaries of the foramen when viewed from the outside looking toward the spinal canal (large arrow) reveal the walls, roof, and floor as depicted in *B*. *(C)* The mixed nerve (s, the sensory portion; m, the motor portion). The relationship of the sensory fibers to the posterior articulations and the relationship of the motor fibers to joints of von Luschka and intervertebral disk are shown.

foramina. Contrary to the motor (anterior) nerve roots, the sensory roots lie at the bottom of the intervertebral foramen and thus may slide below the deformed uncus and escape damage from the osteophyte in neck movement.

The commonest nerve root involvement occurs at the C_6 and C_7 levels, causing paresthesia and pain radiating along the radial side of the arm into the fingers. It is at this site of the cervical spine (C-7) that the greatest degree of motion occurs. It has also been reported (Frykholm) that extension movement of the neck reduces the transverse diameter of the intervertebral foramen, thus causing further encroachment upon the contained nerve roots.

The length of the spinal canal becomes shortened when there is significant multiple disk degeneration. The shortening of the spinal canal changes the site of emergence of the nerve roots. The nerve roots that leave the cord (via their fila) at an angle have a diminution of this angle, and by emerging at a lesser angle, they may emerge at a level lower than normal. Deformation of the cervical spine contour and/or length thus may involve a nerve root higher than its normal level of emergence.

Cervical lordosis is also often altered in cases of spondylosis, and changes in curvature, in length of the spinal canal, and in all the relationships of the nerve roots to their specific foramina may result. This partly explains the difficulty in ascertaining the exact intervertebral or specific root level of many patients' problems.

Nerve-Root Pathology

That nerve-root function is impaired when entrapped by an osteophyte within a diminished foraminal opening is apparent, but the specific tissue changes occurring within the nerve root that lead to symptoms currently remain unclear. Studies (Holt and Yates) reveal that there were changes in the shape of the entrapped, compressed, or stretched ganglia and nerve roots. Histologically these nerve roots were found to have a diffuse increase in the fibrous tissue of the endoneurium (Fig. 8–10). This increased fibrous tissue created a dense network of fibrous tissue separating the individual neurons. With continuing irritation from compression and/or traction, the nerve roots revealed a diminution of the number of neurons and a proliferation of Schwann cells.

There also was noted swelling and fragmentation of the myelin sheaths. The microscopic view of the involved nerve roots show disintegration of the myelin and an irregular ballooned appearance of the root. Many studies reveal the presence of cystic cavities in the nerve roots and the ganglia. These cysts apparently contain cerebrospinal fluid, because they appear to be diverticula of the arachnoid space. The presence of these cysts may also explain why coughing, sneezing, or straining, which elevates cerebrospinal fluid, so frequently increases the symptoms of radiculitis. Hoyland and associates have postulated that encroachment of the intervertebral foramen may cause venous obstruction that may cause mechanical compression of the nerve initially and ultimately lead to

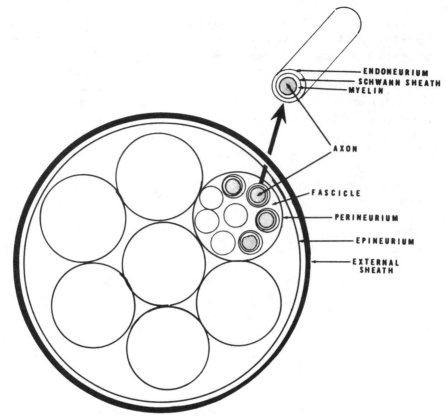

Figure 8–10. Peripheral nerve (schematic). In cross section a nerve is composed of many axons grouped into a fascicle. Each axon is surrounded by myelin enclosed within a sheath of Schwann. This is, in turn, coated with endoneurium, which is composed of longitudinal collagen strips. Perineurium binds the fascicles, which are bound together by epineurium. The entire nerve is covered by an external sheath.

fibrosis.

It remains a matter of conjecture how soon and how reversible these nerve root changes are, but this documentation would be very important in predicting the prognosis following clinical management of cervical spondylosis with radicular signs and symptoms. Obviously early appropriate treatment and careful, frequent, neurologic monitoring of such a patient is mandatory.

As it has been documented that in sensory radicular symptoms neither an EMG nor nerve conduction time findings are of diagnostic or prognostic value (Waylonis), a thorough clinical neurologic evaluation is mandatory.

Cervical spondylosis also effects the width of the spinal canal as well as the width, height, and shape of the intervertebral foramina. This narrowing of the spinal canal, termed *stenosis*, (Fig. 8–11) has the potential to cause cord compression as well as to enhance further nerve-root embarrassment.

The spinal cord fills four fifths of the spinal canal and is held in a taut manner by the dentate ligament (ligamentum denticulatum). This ligament is a broad band of pia mater projecting as a longitudinal fin from each side of the cord. It lies between the ventral and dorsal roots and attaches laterally to the

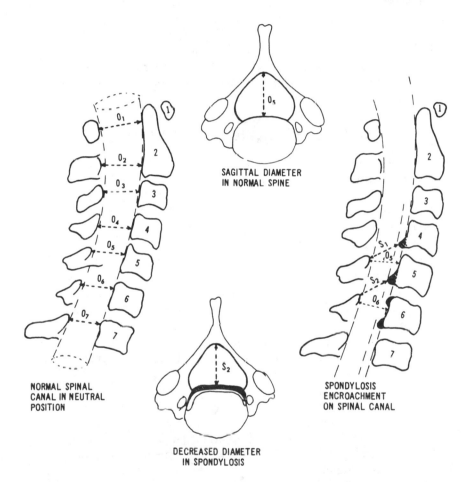

Figure 8–11. Sagittal diameter of the cervical spinal canal. From x-ray studies, the lateral view depicts the sagittal (anteroposterior) diameter of the cervical boney canal. In the neutral position of the normal spine, O_1 averages 22 mm; O_2, 20 mm; and C-3 to C-7 are constant between 12 and 22 mm (average 17 mm). Neck extension from full flexion may alter the diameter by 2 mm. Spondylosis narrows the canal diameter (S_1 and S_2). This measurement is from the posterior border of one vertebra to the upper border of the next lower laminal junction the posterior process. Cord compression may occur if the diameter is 10 mm or less but is improbable if it is 13 mm or more. See text.

dura mater which lines the bony canal. This ligament limits excessive motion of the cord within the canal.

Any encroachment into the canal—such as a bulging intervertebral disk, osteophyte, cyst, tumor, or abscess—can cause compression upon the cord or distraction of the cord because of the dentate ligament. Cord involvement causes cord myelopathy, with upper motor neuron signs and symptoms. This will be thoroughly discussed in the next chapter. It is sufficient to state that any clinical examination of a patient with radiculopathy symptoms and radiologic spondylosis must include the eliciting of hyperactive reflexes and Hoffmann and/or Babinski signs and the determining of neurogenic bowel or bladder symptoms.

The presence of stenosis also mechanically aggravates nerve-root pathology because this narrowing prevents escape of nerve roots under pressure or tension.

DIAGNOSIS AND TREATMENT OF SYMPTOMATIC SPONDYLOSIS

Radicular symptoms, especially in an older person, invoke the possibility of nerve root entrapment from spondylosis. Symptoms consist of numbness or tingling in the thumb, fingers, forearm, upper arm, shoulder, or between the shoulder blades. The subjective complaints of dermatomal distribution are confirmed by careful sensory examination with cotton stroking or light pin scratch.

Often the neck has subjective and objective limited movement. Extension, flexion, lateral flexion, and rotation must be tested, then performed and *held* at their extreme ends of range of motion for brief periods of time to determine whether they reproduce the radicular symptoms in the upper extremity. Most often extension, lateral flexion, or the combination of both reproduces the radicular symptoms.

Motor testing of each upper extremity myotome must also be done. Although sensory loss is most prevalent and often the only deficit, motor impairment must be ascertained.

Upon deducting that there is nerve root involvement, complete radiologic studies must be performed to evaluate the presence, degree, and level of spondylosis. Oblique radiograms as well as lateral views must be taken (1) to establish the status of the zygapophyseal (facet) joints, (2) to determine the level of this change, and (3) to determine the size, contour, and shape of changes in the intervertebral foramina.

An MRI or a CT scan may be of value, but usually a thorough clinical examination and routine x-ray studies suffice to confirm the diagnosis. The possibility that the nerve root signs and symptoms are due to a disk rather than to osteophytes is of academic value inasmuch as both are treated in similar ways.

Response to treatment is also diagnostic *if* the treatment is physiologically appropriate. The following aspects of treatment are similar to those advocated in treating the acute, subacute, and chronic neck disk syndromes discussed in Chapter 7:

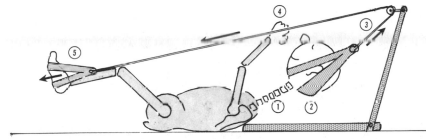

Figure 8–12. Supine cervical traction. This method of cervical traction is applicable at home where it can be applied for a 20-minute period several times a day. Hot packs to the neck can be applied simultaneously. (1) The neck angle (adjustable) allows distraction in slight flexion. (2) The halter pressure is applied to the occiput rather than under the mandible. (3) The angle of traction can be adjusted to the patient's comfort. (4) The hand may apply the traction, adjust the line of pull, and afford security to the patient. (5) Traction is applied by one or both feet, according to the tolerance of the patient.

1. Restore physiologic posture
   a.   Decrease the forward-head posture
   b.   Decrease excessive lordosis
2. Instructions in exercises, ADL, and traction
3. Supine traction with the angle, force, and duration of traction determined by the tolerance and response reaction of the patient (Fig. 8–12)
4. Neck brace or custom-fitted collar to restrict motion and to ensure proper posture. Either of these should be used for sufficient length of time to assure diminution of inflammation but not so long as to cause dependence or disuse
5. Avoidance of any movement that causes or aggravates the radicular symptoms
6. Avoidance of excessive range of motion exercises
7. Judicious use of oral anti-inflammation medicine, antidepressants (if indicated and considered to contribute to excessive pain and to influence the posture)
8. Modification of ADL considered to be aggravating

BIBLIOGRAPHY

Bourdillion, JF: Spinal manipulation. Appleton-Century-Crofts, New York, 1970.

Brain, L: Some unsolved problems of cervical spondylosis. Br Med J March 23, 1930, p 771.

Brain, WR, Knight, GC, and Bull, JWD: Discussion of the intervertebral disk in the cervical region. Proc R Soc Med 41:509, 1948.

Brewerton, DA, et al: Pain in the neck and arm: A multicentre trial of the effects of physiotherapy. Arranged by the British Association of Physical Medicine. Br Med J 29:254, 1966.

Brieg, A and Ahmad, FEN: Biomechanics of the cervical spinal cord. Acta Radiol (Diagn) 4.602, 1966.

Caldwell, JW and Krusen, EM: Effectiveness of cervical traction in treatment of neck problems: Evaluation of various methods. Arch Phys Med Rehabil 43:214, 1962.

Colachis, SC and Strohm, BR: Radiographic studies of cervical spine motion in normal subjects: Flexion and hyperextension. Arch Phys Med Rehabil 46:753, 1965.

Colachis, SC and Strohm, BR: Cervical traction: Relationship of traction time to varied traction forces with constant angle of pull. Arch Phys Med Rehabil 46:815, 1965.

Colachis, SC and Strohm, BR: A study of tractive forces and angle of pull on vertebral interspaces in the cervical spine. Arch Phys Med Rehabil 46:820, 1965.

Collins, DH: The pathology of articular and spinal diseases. Edward Arnold, London, 1949.

Epstein, NE, Epstein, JA, and Carras, R: Cervical spondylosis, stenosis and myeloradiculopathy in patients over 65. Neuro-arthopedics 6:13, 1988.

Fisher, SV, et al: Cervical orthosis effect on cervical spine motion: Roentgenographic and goniometric method of study. Arch Phys Med Rehabil 58:109, 1977.

Friedenberg, ZB and Miller, WT: Degenerative disc disease of the cervical spine. J Bone Joint Surg 45-A, 1171, 1963.

Frykholm, R: Cervical nerve root compression resulting from disc degeneration and root sleeve fibrosis. Acta Chirurgica Scandinavica (Suppl. 160) 1951.

Gregorius, FK, Estrin, T, and Crandall, PH: Cervical spondylotic radiculopathy and myelopathy: A long term follow-up study. Arch Neurol 33:618, 1976.

Hartman, JT, Palumbo, F, and Hill, BJ: Cineradiography of braced normal cervical spine: Comparative study of five commonly used cervical orthoses. Clin Orthrop 109:97, 1975.

Holt, S and Yates, PO: Cervical spondylosis and nerve root lesions. J Bone Joint Surg 48-B(3):407, 1966.

Horwitz, T: Degenerative lesions in the cervical portion of the spine. Arch Intern Med 65, 1178-91, 1940.

Hoyland, JA, Freemont, AJ, and Jayson, M: Intervertebral foramen venous obstruction: a cause of periradicular fibrosis. Spine 14:6, 1988.

Jones, MD: Cineradiographic studies of collar-immobilized cervical spine. J Neurosurg 17:633, 1960.

Jones, MD: Cineradiographic studies of the normal cervical spine. California Medicine 93:293, 1960.

Judavitch, BD: Herniated cervical disc: A new form of traction therapy. Am J Surg 84:646, 1962.

Maroudas, A and Stockwell, RA: Factors involved in the nutrition of the human lumbar intervertebral disc: cellularity and diffusion of glucose in vitro. J Anat 120:113, 1975.

Nathan, H: Osteophytes of the vertebral column. J Bone Joint Surg 44-A:243, 1962.

Odom, GL, Finney, W, and Woodhall, B: Cervical disc lesions. JAMA 166:23, 1958.

Orofino, C, Sherman, MS, and Schechter, D: Luschka's joint: A degenerative phenomenon. J Bone Joint Surg 42-A:853, 1960.

Schmorl, G and Junghanns, H: The human spine in health and disease, ed. 2. Grune and Stratton, New York, 1971.

Symonds, C: The inter-relation of trauma and cervical spondylosis in compression of the cervical cord. Lancet 1:451, 1953.

Tapiovaara, J and Heinevaara, A: Correlation of cervicobrachialgia and roentgenographic findings. Ann Chir Gynecol Fenn (Suppl) 43:436, 1954.

Valtowen, EJ and Kiuro, E: Cervical traction as a therapeutic tool. Scand J Rehabil Med 2:29, 1970.

Vernon-Roberts, B: Disc pathology and disease state. In Ghosh, P (ed): The Biology of the Intervertebral Disc, Vol 11. CRC Press, Boca Raton, FL, 1988.

Vernon-Roberts, B and Pirie, CJ: Degenerative changes in the intervertebral discs of the lumbar spine and their sequelae. Rheumatol Rehabil 16:13, 1977.

Waylonis, GW: Electromyographic findings in chronic cervical radicular syndromes. Arch Phys Med Rehabil. July 1968, 407.

CHAPTER 9

Cervical Spondylotic Myelopathy (CSM)

Cervical spondylosis compressing the spinal cord and causing myelopathy was revealed to the medical public by Brain, Northfield, and Wilkinson in 1952. Prior to that report, many obscure neurologic cord disorders in older people were attributed to undefined "degenerative changes of the central nervous system." With the high frequency of degenerative spondylotic changes in human beings, this revelation accounted for the many central nervous system conditions noted in the elderly.

Considered to be an almost inevitable consequence of aging, osteoarthritis affects nearly 10 percent of the population past the age of 60. This degenerative condition accounts for many painful disabling medical conditions of the peripheral skeletal system and the axial spinal system. Osteoarthritis causing cervical spondylosis was recognized as a degenerative change affecting neck motion and as a cause of local pain and root entrapment syndromes. The article by Brain, Northfield, and Wilkinson alerted the medical profession to its relationship to cord symptoms.

A recent review article in the *New England Journal of Medicine* (Hamerman) has reviewed the current research of the biology of osteoarthritis. It appears that there are changes in the proteoglycans and collagen fibers of cartilage which are now traceable and which may explain the etiology and sequence of ultimate degenerative joint changes. There are also superimposed external forces upon cartilage that contribute to degeneration, such as genetic factors. These changes have not uniformly applied to the intervertebral disk or the cartilage of the zygapophyseal joints, but the sequelae of these changes and spondylosis are being documented. The possibility of genetic and chemical changes has not refuted the factors of trauma, faulty movement, and faulty posture as aggravation of the spondylosis.

The extent, progression, and manifestation of cervical spondylotic myelopathy (CSM) are still unfolding. The prevailing evidence implies that the mechanism of cord damage is from compression of the cord (Nurick). This compression occurs from osteophytes in the anterior portion of the functional unit, degenerative cartilage changes in the posterior zygapophyseal joints, and, often, a predisposed congenital narrowing of the spinal canal.

Intervertebral disk protrusion in an otherwise degenerated spondylotic spine may be the compressive force in CSM. Acute cord compression from an acute angulation of the spine may result in cord compression in a cervical spine with disk degenerative disease. Acute or sustained hyperextension of the neck from an injury, a dental procedure, or a postural position may be the inciting force. Posttraumatic injury may cause vertebral subluxation which may compromise the spinal cord.

The symptoms of myelopathy often begin insidiously and progress slowly. There need not be associated radicular (root) involvement or a firm relationship in the degree of CSM with the degree of noted spondylosis. A gradual onset of CSM may occur with no radiculitis and with minimal x-ray evidence of degenerative changes. Conversely, there may be severe degenerative spinal changes with no central nervous system involvement or impairment. The presence of radicular (root) symptoms often leads to studies that result in finding obscure subtle signs and symptoms of CSM with long tract signs.

Common signs and symptoms of CSM are gait disturbance, impaired fine hand movement, and lower extremity weakness. Findings of spasticity in both the upper and the lower extremities may be discovered during the examination even though significant functional subjective symptoms have not been noted by the patient. Pain is usually not prevalent unless there are associated conditions of root involvement from foraminal stenosis that complement the spinal stenosis.

It must be noted that other conditions mimicking CSM include multiple sclerosis, amyotrophic lateral sclerosis, and syringomyelia, and the encroachment upon the cord causing CSM may be intrinsic or metastatic tumor, abscess, or cyst. A careful differential diagnosis must be clarified before all the signs and symptoms of CSM are attributed to spondylitic spinal stenosis.

In addition to structural spinal cord changes compressing the cord and causing CSM, movement also may be a causative factor. Movement obviously affects any encroachment upon the cord (Brieg and Ahmed) (Fig. 9–1). This factor can be determined by careful history and examination.

The normal spinal canal in the midcervical region is oval, with an average sagittal diameter of 10 mm and width of 17 mm. The cervical cord at this level has a maximum sagittal diameter of 10 mm in the adult. The sagittal diameter of the canal normally increases with neck flexion and decreases with neck extension (Hoff). The canal, and also the foramina as previously stated, may have its opening narrowed by diskogenic changes, posttraumatic angulation, or sub-

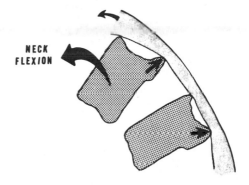

Figure 9–1. Spinal canal stenosis on neck flexion. In cervical spine forward flexion in the presence of spondylosis (osteophytic spurs), the cord and its dural sheath are subjected to traction and compression, thus decreasing the width of the canal.

luxation. In patients who develop CSM there has been noted a greater percentage of people with spinal stenosis (Brain, Northfield, and Wilkinson; Bradley and Banna).

Superimposed upon structural changes is the fact that the opening is also altered by neck motion or posture. Both in flexion and in extension there may be a folding of the ligamentum flavum (Taylor, 1964), which further encroaches upon the contents of the spinal canal (Fig. 9–2).

Damage to the spinal cord, and thus symptoms therefrom, depend upon the specific tract or tracts of the cord involved (Fig. 9–3). Whether cord damage occurs from direct mechanical pressure or from intrinsic cord vascular impairment remains a moot question. Both probably play a significant role.

The spinal cord receives its arterial blood supply from the anterior spinal artery and the paired posterolateral arteries (Fig. 9–4). The anterior spinal artery receives its supply from radicular arteries which originate from the vertebral arteries and deep cervical blood vessels. The anterior spinal artery is usually a single vessel contained in the middle groove of the cord. At its upper level it is formed from a Y bifurcation of the vertebral arteries (Fig. 9–5).

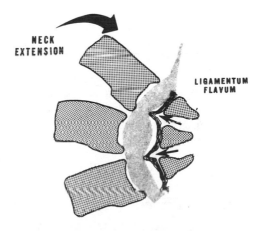

Figure 9–2. Spinal canal stenosis on neck extension. The spinal canal width may be further narrowed by neck extension due to the pleating of the ligamentum flavum.

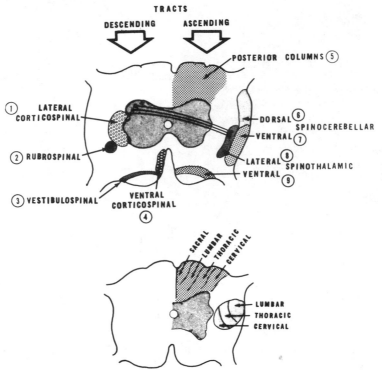

Figure 9–3. Sensory and motor tracts of the spinal cord *(top)*. Generally, the descending tracts (1,2,3,4) are motor, or for coordination, and the ascending tracks (5,6,7,8,9) carry sensation from the periphery to the higher centers. The ascending tracts convey the sensations of pain, touch, proprioception, and discrimination for interpretation *(bottom)*. Areas of the extremities, conveyed by the ascending (dotted area) and descending (lumbar, thoracic, and cervical) tracts.

The anterior spinal artery supplies the central gray area of the cord and the anterolateral white matter. Small branches continue from this artery to join branches of the paired posterior spinal arteries, but they are apparently insufficient to supply adequate blood to the cord in the event of an anterior spinal artery occlusion. The posterior spinal arteries proceed on a circuitous path and are not subjected to traction in neck flexion.

The vascular supply of the cord, the propensity for anterior spinal artery occlusion, and the involvement of the cord area supplied explain the neurologic symptoms and why the anterior columns and outer half of the posterior columns are spared.

The pathologic changes in the cord noted from compression of the anterior spinal artery are in that region of the cord. In a controlled study (Crandall and Gregorious), involvement of the motor system was noted in all cord-involved

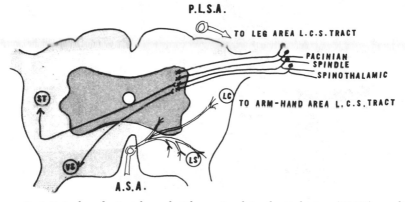

P.L.S.A.

TO LEG AREA L.C.S.TRACT

PACINIAN
SPINDLE

SPINOTHALAMIC

TO ARM-HAND AREA L.C.S.TRACT

A.S.A.

Figure 9–4. Spinal cord arterial supply. The posterolateral spinal artery (PLSA) supplies the lateral corticospinal (LCS) tract to the leg area. The anterior spinal artery (ASA) supplies the region of the cord that contains the lateral corticospinal tract of the arm-hand area. The sensory roots entering the cord contain fibers from end organs within the extremities.

patients with corticospinal tract and spinothalamic tract involvement. It is of interest that during a laminectomy the cord can be seen to blanch from flexion of the neck. Obviously, compression of the cord and sharp angulation of the spinal canal from neck movement are factors that impair cord blood supply with resultant myelopathy, especially in the central gray area and the anterolateral white matter (Hoff).

SYMPTOMS OF CSM

Symptoms of cord involvement in cervical spondylosis usually are subtle and variable. Often the symptoms are not experienced or related by the patient unless ascertained by a careful history and physical examination.

The initial complaint may be an unsteady gait, a feeling of numbness in the trunk, or weakness in the legs or arms. Atrophy of the intrinsic muscles of the hand may be noted, implicating root involvement as well as cord entrapment. Spasticity, which may have been unnoticed or ignored by the patient, may be elicited during the examination.

Pain is usually not significant unless there are related nerve root entrapment symptoms. In cord involvement there may be a feeling of discomfort in the arms, hands, legs, or trunk. Hypersensitivity of the hands and/or feet may be experienced. Impairment of temperature sensation, sense of vibration, or proprioception may not have been a concern of the patient but may become apparent during the examination. "Clumsiness" of the hands and fingers may be the result of spinothalamic cord involvement. Bladder sphincter disturbance

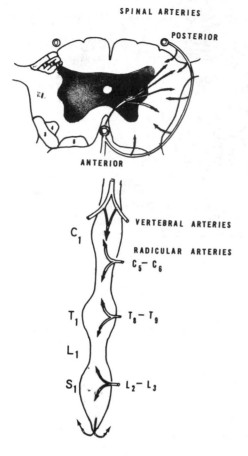

SPINAL ARTERIES

POSTERIOR

ANTERIOR

VERTEBRAL ARTERIES

RADICULAR ARTERIES

C_1

$C_5 - C_6$

T_1

$T_8 - T_9$

L_1

S_1

$L_2 - L_3$

Figure 9–5. Spinal arterial supply *(top)*. The areas of the spinal cord that are supplied by the posterior and anterior spinal arteries are shown. Areas, 1,2A,2B, and 2C are the sensory areas of the Lissauer tracts and the substantia gelatinosa. Areas 3, 4, and 5 are the spinothalamic, spinocerebellar, and corticospinal tracts *(bottom)*. The major radicular arterial branches of the spinal arteries are shown.

may be the first and only symptom experienced by the patient.

It appears that many cord symptoms are noted *after* determining that there is cord involvement. The revelation of neurologic signs of cord involvement leads to a retrospective analysis of symptoms that the patient may have had. It may be that they were relatively minor, were of no great functional loss, or were attributed to the neck and upper extremity symptoms of radiculopathy.

Further documentation of the ambiguity of symptoms that may be experienced by patients and that ultimately may prove to be sequelae of cervical spondylosis is a study by Longfitt and Elliot in which it was noted that "the earliest symptoms of cervical cord compression may be aching in the low back and pain down the legs with no pain or stiffness in the neck." Once cervical spinal stenosis was determined, a laminectomy decompression totally relieved the low back and leg symptoms.

Progression of long tract signs and symptoms may be slow or even unnoticed by the patient. Once discovered, the neurologic signs and symptoms must be monitored periodically by a physician to determine progression and resultant functional impairment (Crandall and Gregorius). These facts enforce the need for thorough neurologic examination in any patient who presents with nerve root entrapment or asymptomatic cervical diskogenic disease found on routine x-ray studies of the neck.

PROGNOSIS

There are extraneous factors that influence the choice of treatment and adversely affect the ultimate prognosis regardless of the treatment. These can be listed in part as:

1. Advanced age
2. Neurogenic sphincter dysfunction
3. Lower extremity weakness out of proportion to the degree of spasticity
4. Severe long-standing neurologic deficit
5. Advanced muscle atrophy
6. Significant concurrent medical problems such as diabetes, pulmonary or cardiovascular disease, atherosclerosis, depression, or severe debility

Other osteoarthritic musculoskeletal disabilities may impair functional improvement even after successful improvement of cord compression symptoms.

EXAMINATION

A careful neurologic examination determines the normalcy of all dermatomes and myotomes of the upper cervical dorsal nerve roots. This examination documents the involvement or the lack of involvement of the nerve roots, following which laboratory tests confirm the adequacy of the foramina. A *functional* examination also confirms the effect of motion upon the nerve roots by extending, flexing, and rotating the neck to reproduce radicular symptoms.

The evaluation of upper motor neuronal impairment from cord compression requires:

1. Eliciting hyperactive tendon reflexes of both the upper and lower extremities
2. Eliciting positive Hoffman and Babinski signs and testing for the Lhermitte sign
3. Observing the gait to determine whether it is spastic or ataxic
4. Testing long tracts carrying proprioception sense (Muscle, Joint, Tendon, vibration, and light touch)
5. Testing for the Romberg sign

LABORATORY CONFIRMATION

Routine spinal x-ray examinations of the cervical spine cast a suspicion of significant disk degeneration, presence and extent of osteophytes and their level, significant degenerative changes of the zygapophyseal joints on oblique views, narrowed or irregular foramina, and a diminished spinal canal width (Fig. 9–6). Subluxation of a vertebra can also be noted, and lateral views of flexion-extension films (Fig. 9–7) may reveal subluxation of a vertebra.

When determining the *pathologic* width of the spinal canal, it must be remembered that the spinal canal width averages 11.8 mm (9 to 15 mm) at the axis (C-2), but at this level osteophytes do not occur. Myelopathy occurs at this level when the width is less than 17.2 mm. Merely finding a narrow canal does not imply cord compression, but it does reveal a predisposition to myelopathy when other conditions such as osteophytes, plicated dura, or subluxation coincide.

Lateral films with flexion-extension views reveal segmental abnormalities of motion and may reveal presence and degree of subluxation not noted on routine static views.

In previous decades myelography alone could reveal the presence, degree, and level of narrowing of the spinal canal. The original Pantopaque has been replaced with soluble dyes or the use of air. This diagnostic procedure is still used by many neurosurgeons to confirm the status of cord compression and to verify its extent and level.

Currently the x-ray examination and myelography have been supplanted or supplemented by CT scanning and MRI. They reveal the most, are easiest to interpret, and, therefore, are most diagnostically effective. Preference varies with the neurosurgical specialist and the neuroradiologist. Both CT scan and MRI are very successful in determining spinal stenosis, foraminal stenoses and their levels, which tissue is responsible, and the extent of stenosis.

Regardless of the accuracy of any laboratory procedure, each of these tests merely documents and confirms the presence and degree of spinal stenosis, but the clinical story and neurologic examination remain the basis of accurate diagnosis.

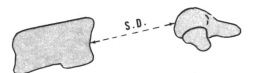

Figure 9–6. Spinal canal width. In measuring the anteroposterior width of the spinal canal, the spinal diameter (SD) is the distance between the posterior margin of the vertebral body and the anteriormost margin of the lamina and zygapophyseal joint.

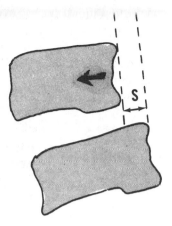

Figure 9–7. Measurement of subluxation. The extent of subluxation *(S)* can be measured by comparing the hindmost protrusion of the vertebral body projecting into the spinal canal with the similar protrusion of an adjacent vertebral body.

TREATMENT

Whether to surgically decompress the myelopathy or treat the patient conservatively remains conjectural. "Conservative therapy still remains a viable therapeutic alternative, . . . although conservative therapy may not stop further deterioration, 30 to 40 percent [of patients] become stable and . . . demonstrate spontaneous improvement" (Roberts).

There have been significant favorable benefits reported from surgical decompression indicating that any patient showing progressive neurologic deficit who is determined to be an otherwise favorable candidate, should have the option of surgical decompression.

Success or failure of surgery cannot be predicted by specific preoperative findings, but it is an accepted fact that preoperative bladder dysfunction and marked lower extremity weakness are unfavorable prognostic factors. Even with successful surgical decompression, many patients continue to progress in their neurologic deterioration. Surgical procedures cannot be thoroughly discussed in this text as they are too numerous and each is complex. The procedures vary from posterior decompression with or without fusion or anterior interbody decompression and fusion. Many favor the latter insofar as postoperative subluxation is minimized, which, when present, portends further cord compression.

CONSERVATIVE TREATMENT

Insofar as increased lordosis and forward-head posture shorten the cervical spinal canal, the main objective is to lengthen the canal by treatment modalities. Inasmuch as movement, especially excess movement, imposes traction and friction upon the embarrassed cord, prevention of excess motion is indicated.

Prevention of excess passive motion from external forces strengthening the neck musculature is also indicated. A collar adds protection to an excess external force, but strong musculature insures it to a greater degree. Recommend that the patient's activities of daily living be modified to avoid sustained postures of excess extension, rotation, lateral flexion, or a combination. Dental visits must be limited as should activities about the house (i.e., working overhead).

All of the above treatments have been discussed in previous chapters but a summary is warranted:

1. Traction in cervical spondylosis with myelopathy has not been proven to be of great value
2. A molded custom fitted collar or brace is probably the most effective treatment. This may be the Philadelphia brace, SOMI Brace, a fiberglass molded brace, or one of many others on the market. They must immobilize the head and neck and hold the head directly above the cervical spine; *chin-in* posture insures a diminished lordosis and will minimize neck motion in all directions.
3. Exercises to strengthen the neck short flexors and long extensors
4. Avoidance of excessive attempts to increase range of motion
5. Avoidance of manipulation
6. Instruct patient in proper postures during the day, modification of faulty postures and positions during ADL ("neck school").
7. Judicious use of oral anti-inflammatory medicine and endorphin enhancers

BIBLIOGRAPHY

Adams, CBT and Lague, V: Studies in cervical spondylotic myelopathy, III: Some functional effects of operations for cervical spondylotic myelopathy. Brain 94:587, 1971.

Bradley, WG and Banna, M: The cervical dural canal: A study of the "tight dural canal" and syringomyelia by prone and supine myelopathy. Br J Radiol 41:608, 1968.

Bradshaw, P: Some aspects of cervical spondylosis. Q J Med 26:177, 1957.

Brain, L: Some unsolved problems of cervical spondylosis. Br Med J March 23, 1963, 771.

Brain, WR, Northfield, DW, and Wilkinson, M: The neurological manifestations of cervical spondylosis. Brain 75:187, 1952.

Brieg, A and Ahmed, FEN: Biomechanics of the cervical spinal cord. Acta Radiol (Diagn) 4:602, 1966.

Brieg, A and Turnbull, HO: Effects of mechanical stresses on the spinal cord in cervical spondylosis: A study of fresh cadaver material. J Neurosurg 25:45, 1966.

Bucy, PC, Heimberger, RF, and Aberhill, HR: Compression of the cervical spinal cord by herniated intervertebral discs. J Neurosurg 5:471, 1948.

Burrows, EH: The sagittal diameter of the spinal canal in cervical spondylosis. Clin Radiol 14:77, 1963.

Chakravorty, BG: Arterial supply of the cervical spinal cord and its relation to the cervical myelopathy in spondylosis. Ann R Coll Surg Engl 45:232, 1969.

Clark E and Robinson, PK: Cervical myelopathy: A complication of cervical spondylosis. Brain 79:483, 1956.

Collins, DH: The pathology of articular and spinal diseases. Edward Arnold, London, 1949.

Crandall, PH and Gregorius, FK: Long term followup of surgical treatment of cervical spondylotic myelopathy Spine 2(2):139, 1977.

Epstein, NE, Epstein, JA, and Carras, R: Cervical spondylosis, stenosis and myeloradiculopathy in patients over 65: Diagnostic techniques and management. Neuro-orthopedic 6:16, 1988.

Gregorius, FK, Estrin, T, and Crandall, PH: Spondylotic radiculopathy and myelopathy. Arch Neurol 33:618, 1976.

Hamerman, D: The biology of osteoarthritis. N Engl J Med. May 18, 1989, 1322.

Hoff, J, et al: The role of ischemia in the pathogenesis of cervical spondylotic myelopathy. Spine 2:2, 1977.

Holt, S and Yates, PO: Cervical spondylosis and nerve root lesions. J Bone Joint Surg 48B(3):407, 1966.

Longfitt, TW and Elliott, FA: Pain in the low back and legs caused by cervical cord compression. JAMA 200:383, 1967.

Nurick, S: The pathogenesis of the spinal cord disorder associated with cervical spondylosis. Brain 95:87, 1972.

Nurick, S: The natural history and the results of surgical treatment of the spinal cord disorder associated with cervical spondylosis. Brain 95:101, 1972.

Roberts, AH: Myelopathy due to cervical spondylosis treated by collar immobilization. Neurology 16:952, 1966.

Schneider, RC, Cherry, B, and Pantek, H: The syndrome of acute central cervical cord injury with special reference to the mechanics involved in hyperextension injuries of the cervical spine. J Neurosurg 11:546, 1954.

Stookey, B: Compression of the spinal cord and nerve roots by herniation of the nucleus pulposus in the cervical region. Arch Surg 40:417, 1940.

Taylor, AR: Mechanism and treatment of spinal and disorders associated with cervical spondylosis. Lancet 1:717, 1953.

Taylor, AR: Vascular factors in the myelopathy associated with cervical spondylosis. Neurology 14:62, 1964.

Vernon-Roberts, B and Pirie, CJ: Degenerative changes in the intervertebral discs of the lumbar spine and their sequelae. Rheumatol Rehabil, 16:13, 1977.

Waylonis, GW: Electromyographic findings in chronic cervical radicular syndromes. Arch Phys Med Rehabil. July, 1968, 407.

CHAPTER 10

Differential Diagnosis of Neck, Arm, and Hand Pain

Many conditions simulate pain in the neck and the shoulder with feelings of discomfort in the upper extremity—arm, hand, and fingers. Many of these conditions cause pain and paresthesia in dermatomal areas that mimic cervical radicular symptoms and these require differential diagnosis.

A condition of neurovascular compression syndrome of the thoracic outlet was first implied by Thorburn in 1905. The condition gained great importance and was diagnosed frequently at first. It was treated by numerous physical therapeutic modalities and even became a diagnosis requiring surgical intervention. Time has given less credence to the existence of this condition, to the point that many now consider this entity to be neither anatomically possible nor clinically verifiable (Roos; Wilbourn).

Assuming that there is a subjective clinical syndrome of paresthesia and weakness of the upper extremity from neurovascular bundle entrapment in the thoracic outlet, it must be considered in the differential diagnosis of cervical radiculitis as not completely conforming to nerve root entrapment at the foraminal level.

The compression syndromes in the thoracic outlet (TOS) have been termed *scalene anticus syndrome, claviculocostal syndrome,* and *pectoralis minor syndrome,* depending upon which anatomic structure is considered responsible for the compression. There are other diagnostic labels, such as *undisputed axonopathic neurogenic* TOS and disputed "droopy shoulder" TOS (Hall).

The neurovascular structures involved in the outlet are the branches of the brachial plexus (Fig. 10–1), which are composed of the primary anterior rami of C_5, C_6, C_7, C_8, and T_1. The blood vessels are the subclavian artery and subclavian vein.

After emerging from their foramina, the nerve rami (roots) descend and

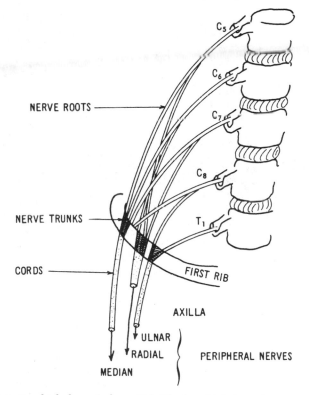

Figure 10–1. Brachial plexus (schematic). The brachial plexus is composed of the anterior primary rami of C_5, C_6, C_7, C_8, and T_1. The roots emerge from the intervertebral foramina through the scalene muscles. The roots merge into three trunks in the region of the first rib. The trunks via divisions become cords that divide into the peripheral nerves of the upper extremities.

are situated between the scalene muscles. They proceed laterally and downward, merging into three trunks (upper trunk, C_5 and C_6; middle trunk, C_7; and lower trunk, C_8 and T_1). They may have an added input from C_4 and T_2.

The trunks divide and pass under the clavicle just lateral to the first rib. These divisions then unite to form the three cords located in the axilla. These three cords give rise to the majority of the peripheral nerves that supply the upper extremity.

The plexus, artery, and vein pass over the top of the first rib in close proximity to the rib. The subclavian vein lies anterior to the scalene anticus muscle which separates it from the nerve fibers (Fig. 10–2). The scalene anticus muscle originates from the cervical vertebrae and attaches to the first rib.

Directly behind the scalene anticus muscle lies the subclavian artery. Lateral to (behind) the artery lies the neurologic bundle, and behind it is the

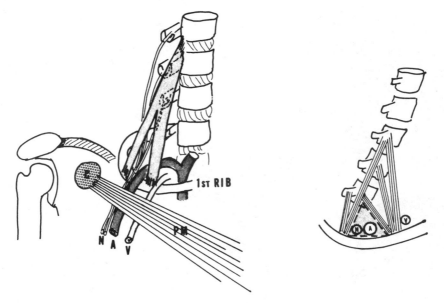

Figure 10–2. The supraclavicular space. The scalene muscles originate from the cervical spine and divide to contain the brachial plexus *(N)* and the subclavian artery *(A)*. The middle scalene muscle is posterior and the anterior scalene muscle is anterior to the artery. The subclavian vein *(V)* is anterior to the anterior scalene muscle. After passing over the first rib (not shown), the neurovascular bundle passes under the smaller pectoral muscle. The clavicle covers the neurovascular bundle and lies parallel to the first rib. The corcoid process is labeled *C*.

scalene medius. The neurovascular bundle (nerve roots and artery) therefore, lies between the anterior and medial scalene muscles and on the first rib (see Fig. 10–2).

The pain syndrome termed TOS implies compression of this neurovascular bundle. Therein also lies the clinical controversy in that many clinical syndromes are neuropathic (sensory) and not vascular. The neuropathic signs and symptoms are paresthesia, as well as pain with numbness and tingling and variable motor deficits.

The symptoms depend on whether the nerves, the blood vessels, or both are compressed. The nerve symptoms are paresthesia, pain, or subjective weakness, whereas the vascular symptoms are edema, pallor, discoloration, or venous congestion.

In syndromes of axonopathic TOS there is objective weakness and wasting of median and ulnar nerve distribution of the hand and forearm. The sensory impairment is usually of the ulnar distribution in the forearm and hand. For some reason the median sensory distribution is spared. Pain, when present, may also be in the dermatomal distribution.

With ulnar distribution myopathy the intrinsics of the hand, including the thenar and hypothenar eminences, are affected. The first dorsal interosseous is involved, and the hand develops the characteristic *hollowed out* appearance. Thumb opposition to the little finger is weak, and there is weakness of spreading the fingers. There may be difficulty in flexing the distal phalanges of the thumb and first finger and flexion of the wrist in an ulnar deviated direction.

Pain, numbness, and tingling are felt in the ulnar aspect of the forearm and the little fingers. Thus subjective complaint can be confirmed by cotton touch and pin scratch.

Confirmatory x-ray studies may reveal a large down-curving transverse process of the seventh cervical vertebra, a rudimentary cervical rib, or a boney abnormality of the clavicle. It must be remembered that a cervical rib is found in 1 percent of normal population and is not diagnostic. A CT scan can clarify boney abnormalities, and arteriography can demonstrate vascular stenosis when vascular symptoms are most prominent and objectively demonstrated. The presence of abnormal boney changes of the thoracic outlet are not confirmation of those changes as the cause of the TOS symptoms.

Electromyographic tests are considered the most confirmatory of TOS. Nerve conduction time studies may reveal the entrapment when the electrical stimulation is at Erb's point and there is delay across the thoracic outlet. An EMG of the involved muscles of the upper extremity may reveal motor nerve involvement. An F wave response has been advocated by electromyographers as being diagnostic. More recently, somatosensory evoked potentials are being evaluated as to their diagnostic specificity.

Because there remain many who favor the clinical diagnosis of TOS and subdivide the syndrome into scalene anticus, claviculocostal, and pectoralis minor syndromes, all three merit consideration. All three essentially present the same symptoms of neurovascular bundle compression, but their anatomic differences are what culminate in the diagnostic labels.

ANTERIOR SCALENE SYNDROME

The symptoms of the anterior scalene syndrome are numbness and tingling of the arm and fingers. Patients describe the paresthesia as "going to sleep" or "pins and needles" of the hands and fingers. There is the complaint of diminished sensation, clumsiness of movement, and weakness. Pain, when claimed, is described as a deep, dull vague aching in the arm and hand.

Many of these symptoms appear during the early morning hours and may awaken the patient. They may also come on after prolonged sitting, especially if these sitting positions are accompanied by manual activities such as knitting or sewing.

Physical findings are usually minimal or absent. Objective vascular changes of swelling, color changes, sweating, hand pallor, or excessive perspiration are rarely found. When found, they portend significant neurovascular pathology. Objective neurologic signs, including atrophy and loss of deep tendon reflex, also are rarely found. Sensory *loss*, meaning diminished sense of light touch of pin prick or cotton, is subjective and not always strictly dermatomal.

A positive diagnostic test result has been attributed to eliciting the Adson test, or the so-called anterior scalene test. This test is performed by turning the head to the side of the involved extremity and simultaneously extending the head, abducting the arm, and taking and holding a deep breath. A positive Adson test result is the reproduction of the symptoms with simultaneous obliteration of the radial pulse in that hand.

Merely to observe obliteration of the radial pulse is not diagnostic of any condition, inasmuch as the pulse is obliterated or diminished in a large number of normal asymptomatic people. Reproduction of the paresthesia suggests the clinical diagnosis of TOS.

The mechanism causing this Adson type of reaction is considered as follows: The anterior scalene muscle originates from the cervical vertebral transverse processes of the third to the sixth vertebrae. It inserts as a broad band into the upper surface of the first rib near the sternum. As the brachial plexus and the subclavian artery pass over the rib, the artery lies posterior to the scalene muscle. Behind the brachial plexus the scalene medius muscle attaches to the rib. The triangle formed by the scalenes provides the opening through which the neurovascular bundle passes.

Turning the head elongates the scalene muscle, as does taking a deep breath (it is an accessory inspiratory muscle), theoretically compressing the bundle which is stretched by abducting the arms (Fig. 10–3).

Why these symptoms occur in otherwise asymptomatic people, usually in an older group, with no structural abnormalities remains conjectural. Spasm of the scalenes may result from usual physical activity, anxiety, tension, or as a residual of external trauma such as a hyperextension injury. Prolonged faulty posture may be causative, hence the diagnostic label of *droopy shoulder syndrome*. All too often no causative factor(s) can be elicited in a careful history.

The forward head posture with increased lordosis (Fig. 10–4) may cause nerve root irritation from closure of the foramina (Fig. 10–5). This irritates the nerve roots and especially the posterior primary division, causing the cervical muscles (including the scalenes) to undergo reactive contraction. The fact that this condition (TOS) occurs in the older age group is also attributable to the presence of diskogenic narrowing (spondylosis) of the foramina in the aging population.

The presence of a cervical rib—an accentuated transverse process of the lowest cervical vertebra—has also been considered the causative mechanical factor in compression of the bundle. This is highly improbable inasmuch as this "rib" has been present throughout the patient's life, thus only contiguous factors *plus* the rib can be given credence. Asymptomatic cervical ribs and TOS occur usually without the presence of a cervical rib, hence the relationship is nebulous.

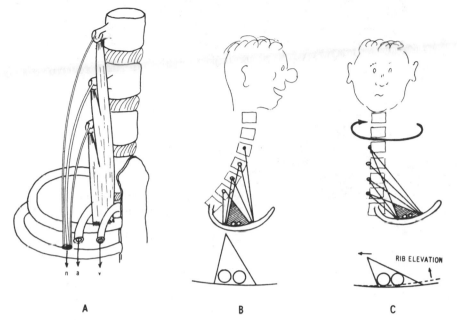

Figure 10–3. Scalene anticus syndrome. *(A)* Relationship of the neurovascular bundle. The subclavian artery *(a)* passes behind the anterior scalene muscle, loops over the first rib, and is joined by the brachial plexus *(n)*. The artery is separated from the subclavian vein *(v)* by the anterior scalene muscle. The median scalene muscle (not shown) lies behind the nerve *(n)*. *(B)* The triangle formed by the scalenes and the first rib. *(C)* Distortion from turning the head toward the symptomatic side. Also, the first rib elevates as a result of deep inspiration, the scalenes being inspiratory muscles. Compression of the neurovascular bundle *(n, a,* and occasionally *v)* can be pictured from the test maneuver of the anticus scalene syndrome.

Treatment of TOS

Treatment for TOS and anterior scalene syndrome is similar to that for cervical diskogenic syndrome:

1. Improve posture (Figs. 10–6, 10–7)
2. Improve ADL aspects of posture (Fig. 10–8)
3. Improve neck flexibility—ROM
4. Judicious use of home traction if the symptoms have significant severity to justify it
5. Use of a cervical collar to enhance posture and to relieve muscular tension until exercise and training become effective
6. Oral medication to enhance muscular relaxation or to overcome depression and anxiety

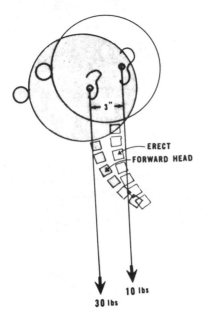

Figure 10–4. Gravity effect upon the cervical spine. With erect posture, the weight of the head (approximately 10 pounds) is held directly above the center of gravity. In a forward-head posture, the head is held inches ahead of the center of gravity and weighs the weight of the head multiplied by the inches ahead of the center: 3" = 30 lb, 4" = 40 lb.

Because many patients with TOS are middle-aged and poorly postured with dorsal kyphosis and weakened shoulder girdle muscles, exercises to strengthen the shoulder girdle muscles are valuable.

These exercises are essentially shoulder shrugging exercises against resistance for strength and, when done repeatedly, for endurance. In the seated position with the neck retracted in a correct posture, the shoulders are elevated slowly, against resistance, to full elevation, held, and then the exercise is repeated. The resistance can be buckets filled with increasing amounts of water, or other similar weights can easily be managed.

The same exercise should be done in the correct standing position. The shoulders are elevated (Figs. 10–9, 10–10), posteriorly retracted, held, and lowered. The exercise is then repeated.

A diagnosis of anterior scalene syndrome mandates that the syndrome of cervical radiculitis or other supraclavicular pathology has been ruled out.

CLAVICULOCOSTAL SYNDROME

Symptomatic thoracic outlet, neurovascular bundle compression, or TOS is also attributed to compression of the bundle between the clavicle (collar bone) and the first rib. Because both bones affect the neurovascular bundle compression, this syndrome is termed *claviculo costal syndrome* (Fig. 10–11). Like TOS, the factors responsible for this syndrome are considered to be faulty

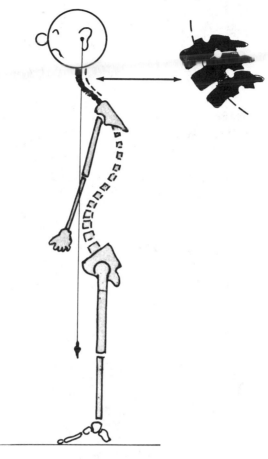

Figure 10–5. Effect of posture upon the cervical spine. The slumped forward posture causes the head to be held ahead of the center of gravity. The cervical spine must assume a greater lordosis to balance and thus closes the intervertebral foramina and places more pressure upon the zygapophyseal (facet) joints.

posture, fatigue, anxiety, and depression, the latter being the cause of the "droopy posture."

The symptoms are the same, namely, numbness, tingling, and weakness of the arms and hands noted principally in the early hours of the morning.

Unlike the anterior scalene syndrome, however, the claviculocostal syndrome often produces a negative Adson test result. The diagnosis is suggested by the obliteration of the pulse and the reproduction of the upper extremity symptoms by bringing the shoulders down and back and holding them there briefly. This scapular motion is done actively by the patient, then passively to the patient.

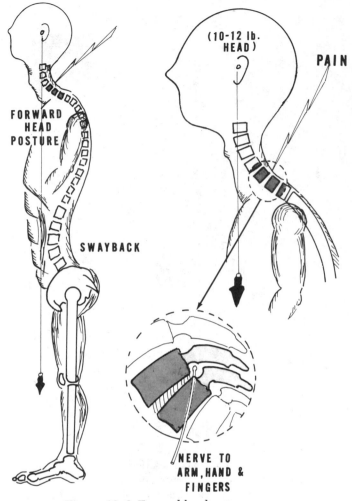

Figure 10–6. Forward-head posture.

Many anatomists have refuted this possibility by demonstrating that it is "anatomically impossible to compress the neurovascular bundle between the clavicle and the first rib." The separation of these two bones and their relationship to the brachial plexus and the subclavian artery essentially justify eliminating this TOS theory.

PECTORALIS MINOR SYNDROME

The pectoralis minor muscle originates from the third, fourth, and fifth

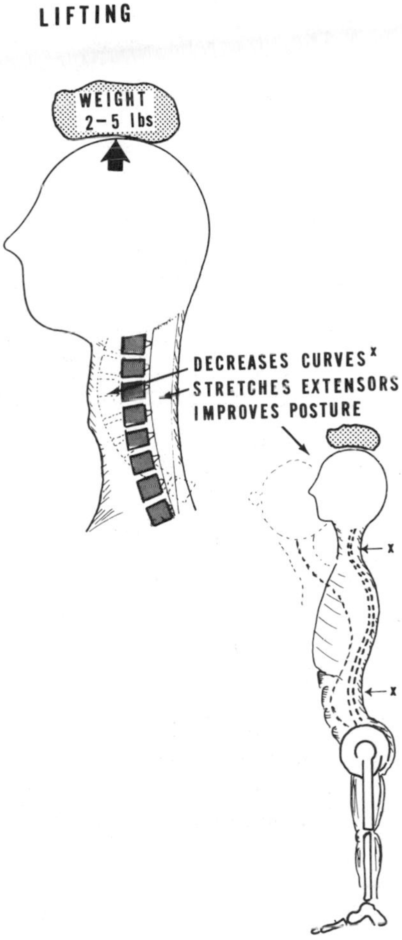

Figure 10–7. Distraction exercise to improve posture.

ribs in the anterior midcostal area and inserts into the coracoid process of the scapula. Occasionally the muscle also originates from the second and/or sixth rib.

The cord division of the brachial plexus descends over the rib cage in the axilla accompanied by the axillary artery and vein, where it is covered by the pectoralis minor muscle. Any neurovascular compression is considered to exist between the rib cage and the overlying pectoralis muscle (see Fig. 10–11, lower portion of *B*).

In this syndrome the symptoms are identical to those in the two syndromes previously discussed, but the diagnostic maneuver is to bring the arms overhead, abduct them, and bring them slightly back. By acquiring this position the pec-

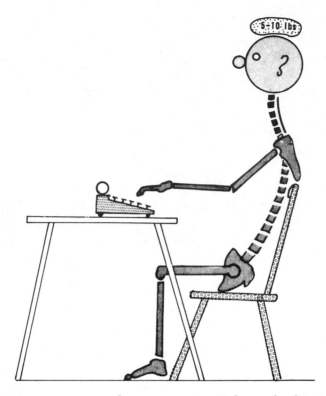

Figure 10–8. Distraction exercise for posture training. With a weight of 5 to 10 lbs within a sandbag upon the head, the posture is maintained erect and the cervical lordosis is minimal. Proprioceptive concept of posture is learned with no effort.

toralis minor muscle stretches and (theoretically) mechanically compresses the neurovascular bundle against the rib cage. This motion and position causes the symptoms as well as obliterates the wrist pulses.

Treatment of this syndrome is similar to that of the others, that is, concentrating on the posture, strengthening the scapular musculature, and gently and gradually stretching the pectoralis muscle. This stretching requires bringing the arms behind the head and gently, frequently, stretching the pectoralis muscles. Faulty posture remains the major culprit.

SCAPULOCOSTAL SYNDROME

Pain between the shoulder blades, which is so often a sequela of the radiculitis of cervical diskogenic disease (Cloward), may also be a muscular com-

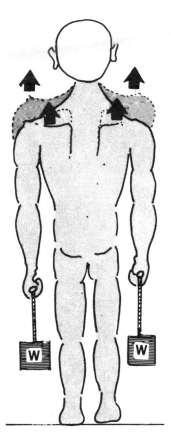

Figure 10–9. Standing scapular elevation exercises. With proper posture (tilted pelvis and flattened cervical lordosis) both arms are rhythmically elevated, held, and slowly lowered. Increasing weights are used. Elbows must be fully extended.

ponent of faulty posture, which has been postulated as a factor in diskogenic disease. This entity must be differentiated in the evaluation of a patient with this complaint.

The *scapulocostal syndrome* is the term applied to the muscular symptoms of persistent dorsal kyphotic *(round back)* posture (Fig. 10–12). Due to the downward gliding of the scapula upon the rib cage with simultaneous outward rotation of the shoulder blade, the muscles that support the blade are placed under persistent sustained muscular contraction and strain. These scapular muscles are primarily the levator scapulae and the rhomboid group as well as fiber of the upper trapezius.

The cause of this muscular syndrome is postural. It becomes evident from prolonged occupational positions, such as those assumed in typing, viewing a computer, using bifocal glasses, and so forth. This posture may also be sustained from chronic fatigue, depression, anger, and anxiety. This syndrome may also be a component of the palpable nodules noted in fibromyositis.

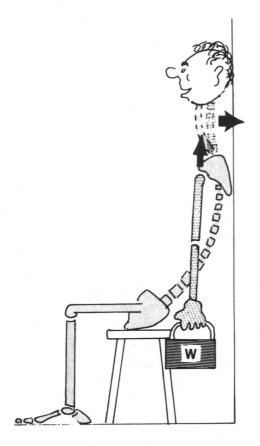

Figure 10–10. Scapular elevation exercises. Patient is seated with back to wall, head and neck pressed against the wall, which decreases the cervical lordosis. With arms fully extended and dependent, weights are lifted in a shrugging motion. Weights vary from 5 to 30 lbs.

The diagnosis of scapulocostal syndrome is a clinical observation, inasmuch as there are no neurologic signs, no laboratory confirmatory tests, and all blood and x-ray study results are negative. Lateral x-ray views of the thoracic spine may confirm the excessive kyphosis. Usually there is also noted a compensatory cervical lordosis and a forward-head posture.

Treatment of Scapulocostal Syndrome

The goal of treatment is essentially (1) treatment of the acute manifestations, (2) prevention of recurrence or aggravation, and (3) prevention of the condition becoming chronic. Because muscular soreness and tenderness are the result of mechanical tension of the scapular muscles with consequential muscular ischemia and inflammation, acute treatment is:

1. Rest of the involved anatomic structures—scapular immobilization is

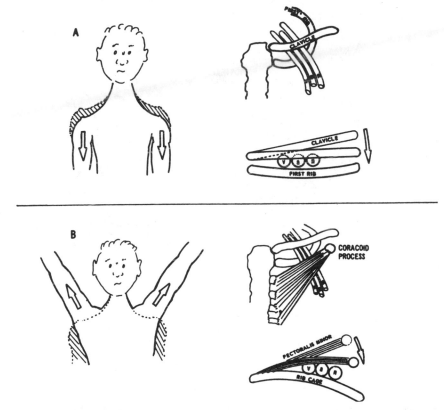

Figure 10–11. Claviculocostal syndrome and pectoralis minor syndrome. *(A)* Claviculocostal syndrome. The neurovascular bundle is compressed between the clavicle and the first rib by retraction and depression of the shoulder girdles. *(B)* Pectoralis minor syndrome. The neurovascular bundle may be compressed between the pectoralis minor and the rib cage by elevating the arms in a position of abduction and moving the arms behind the head.

difficult, but frequently a soft figure 8 bandage decreases the downward rotation of the scapula and adducts (supports) the scapulae, bringing them into midline position toward the thoracic spine
2. Local modalities such as ice packs or vasocoolant sprays for a few days, followed by local heat moist packs, infrared, or ultrasound
3. Deep friction or effleurage massage, followed by passive stretch of the inflamed muscles
4. Oral nonsteroidal anti-inflammatory medication
5. Injection into the sites of deep tenderness and/or nodularity with an anesthetic agent and/or a steroid agent
6. Attention to the posture with training, exercises, modification of ADL

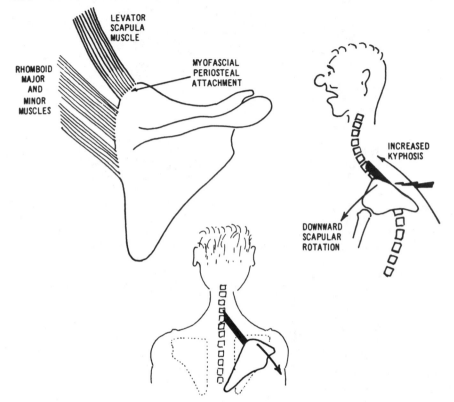

Figure 10–12. Scapulocostal syndrome. Pain located by the patient in the upper inter-scapular area, and surmised to be between the medial border of the shoulder blade and the underlying rib cage, is a myofusio-periostitis. The *trigger area* is the site of attachment of the levator scapula muscle to the upper medial angle of the scapula. The mechanism is postural and tension traction of the attachment site.

7. Cervical traction has limited value but often assists in overcoming the postural component
8. Antidepressant medication and, when applicable, psychologic guidance.

CHRONIC MUSCULOSKELETAL PAIN SYNDROMES

Chronic musculoskeletal pain syndromes (CMPS) with no discernible organic cause of muscle pathology have become a diagnostic and therapeutic challenge to the general population and a dilemma to the medical profession.

Millions of dollars are spent monthly in the diagnostic and therapeutic approaches to this ill-defined entity. Many times diagnosis of CMPS has been a diagnosis of exclusion.

Numerous diagnostic labels have been appended to this condition, such as *fibrositis, fibromyositis, myofascitis, interstitial myofascitis, tension myositis, psychogenic rheumatism, primary fibromyalgia syndrome (PFS)*, and numerous others. Recently there have been attempts to clarify this disease entity, such as those of the Toxonomy Subcommittee of the International Association for the Study of Pain.

Three CMPS classifications have emerged: (1) PFS, (2) myofascial pain syndrome (MPS), and (3) temporomandibular pain and dysfunction syndrome (TMPDS). Admittedly all three interrelate, and there is a direct, albeit vague, relationship among the three.

Primary Fibromyalgia Syndrome

Primary fibromyalgia syndrome has been diagnosed by the following criteria (Yunus):

Obligatory

1. Generalized aches and pains (or stiffness) in at least three anatomic sites for at least three months
2. Absence of traumatic injury, structural rheumatic disease, infectious arthropathy, endocrine-related arthropathy, and abnormal test results.

Major

1. Change in symptoms with activity
2. Change in symptoms with weather
3. Change in symptoms with anxiety or stress
4. Poor sleep
5. General fatigue
6. Anxiety
7. Headache
8. Irritable bowel
9. Subjective swelling
10. Nonradicular, nondermatomal numbness.

Many of these criteria correlate with the diagnostic criteria of Smythe and Moldofsky, who postulate five criteria:

1. Widespread aching for more than 3 months
2. Local tenderness at 12 or 14 specific sites
3. Skin-rolling tenderness over the upper scapular region
4. Disturbed sleep, with morning fatigue and stiffness
5. Normal erythrocyte sedimentation rate (ESR), serum glutamic-oxaloacetic transaminase (SGOT), rheumatoid factor test result, antinuclear factor (ANF), muscle enzymes, and sacroiliac film study results.

Both the obligatory criteria and the first 10 of the major criteria are strictly subjective and are based on exclusion of positive objective test results or signs. It is difficult to document these symptoms objectively and to give an organic diagnosis. To the many physicians who deny the existence of a specific diagnosis of primary fibromyositis and consider all the symptoms to be psychogenic, there is a basis for this assumption.

The criteria of Smythe are more confirmable in that they delineate the sites of muscular tenderness to specific regions before the diagnosis is valid. It is true that tenderness is wholly subjective, even though the dolorimeter has been advocated as objectively documenting and grading the degree of pain from tissue pressure. Psychogenic etiology is thus not negated.

The most specific basis for the presence of PFS (Smythe) is the corroboration of the sleep disturbance postulated by Modolfsky (1975) in his sleep laboratory studies of PFS patients and normal asymptomatic people. The finding of a relationship between PFS and sleep deprivation not only adds credence to the entity existing but also suggests a form of effective treatment via correction of the sleep impairment.

Assuming the presence of PFS, the patient (usually female) presents with diffuse prolonged muscular aching and generalized stiffness. This aching and stiffness occurs primarily in the proximal extremities and, in a given patient, remains in a consistent pattern.

The large majority of patients present tenderness in the shoulder (girdle) region and in the arms. All portions of all extremities and trunk, however, are not immune. Some paresthesia may occur, with subjective swelling of the hands and fingers. The areas of specific sites of tenderness have been well-documented by Yunus and by Smythe.

Therein lies another point of controversy: that of differentiating PFS from MPS. Both present tender nodules and the *jump sign* (Kraft, Johnson, and LeBan) upon pressure and release. Both also have positive skin-rolling tenderness, especially over the upper scapular regions. A differential point to make is that there is distal referral of pain upon pressure of the tender nodule in MPS, whereas the pain in PFS is local and nonradiating.

Treatment of PFS. Treatment of PFS has been reviewed recently (Buckelew) in detail regarding its efficacy and its scientific basis.

The widely accepted treatment of PFS has been:

1. Reassurance (Smythe) based on an explanation of the nature of the disease to the patient. This would be feasible if there could be reassurance to the patient that relief can be expected, disability diminished, and recurrence prevented. Such has not been the experience of most clinicians. To assure the patient that the illness is not ominous is of little benefit. To explain the illness would be possible only if the average physician had an explanation that he or she fully understood and believed.

2. Symptomatic treatment with heat massage, ice, TENS, and so forth is

nonspecific and frequently of limited value with little or no carry over. As placebo therapy for temporary relief it is of value to the patient, provided it is not expensive, addictive, or carried out indefinitely.

3. Physical exercises are probably of the greatest value because these ultimately increase the endorphins (serotonin) in the body. Unfortunately, exercises to the required degree are rarely accepted and undertaken by the patient because they must be of significant duration, must be done with tolerance of some discomfort, and require self-discipline. This is an active type of therapy, and most PFS patients request passive therapy done *to* them, not *by* them.

4. Evaluation of mechanical stressors and emotional stressors. Evaluation of mechanical stressors is extremely valuable but may be difficult to implement in the treatment program. Emotional stressors are difficult to determine, to be accepted by the patient, and usually they are extremely difficult to alter.

5. Use of tricyclics, which are also seratonin enhancers, have been shown to be of value and, as shown by Moldofsky (1980), restore the more physiologic sleep pattern. Because these are mood modifiers, their benefit contributes to the idea that PFS is a psychogenic disease.

6. Psychologic intervention involves biofeedback, operant conditioning, self-hypnosis, counseling, and even psychotherapy. All have many advocates, yet good control studies have yet to determine what long-term value each of these approaches has.

Buckelew's conclusion is that the treatment of PFS is a multidisciplinary rehabilitation approach, but studies to confirm which aspects of a particular discipline will give long-term benefits have been lacking. All methods should be tried with an open mind, but none should be pursued *ad infinitum* when there are insufficient benefits evident.

Myofascial Pain Syndrome

The criteria suggested (McCain and Scudds) to accept the diagnosis of MPS, the second of the considered CMPS, are:

1. Local tenderness at one or a few points in the musculoskeletal system
2. A distinct pattern of referred pain
3. The presence of a taut, palpable band within the tender muscle
4. A local twitch response to quick tapping
5. Associated muscle weakness and limited movement

The presence of palpable active trigger points which refer pain upon being palpated suggests the diagnosis of MPS. These referred sites are not myotomal or dermatomal but supposedly have a specific pattern (Travell and Simons) (Fig. 10–13).

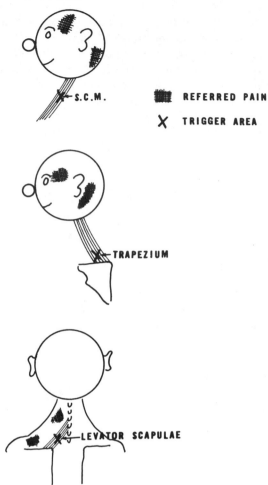

Figure 10–13. Trigger points and referred pain. Tender areas in various part of the neck and shoulder, when irritated, can refer pain to distal sites.

Because there is also the assumption that the conditions of MPS and PFS are psychogenic, studies such as the Minnesota Multiphasic Personality Inventory (MMPI) have found a higher incidence of abnormality in PFS patients than in rheumatoid arthritis patients. Irritable bowel syndrome, sleep disturbance, headaches, and peripheral paresthesia have been well documented in psychologic disease patterns with no accompanying organic disease.

Until more is known about the neurophysiologic relationship of the muscular system to the vegetative emotional conditions, to deny the existence of PFS and merely to assume that these conditions are purely psychologic is redundant. Assuming that the etiology is psychogenic does not minimize or eliminate the debilitating and disabling aspects.

Treatment of the musculoskeletal symptoms of MPS is essentially that advocated by Travell and Simons, namely *stretch and spray* of the involved tender muscle bundles and 0.5 percent procaine injections into palpable trigger sites. Travell and Simons also advocate flexibility exercises, posture training, modifying faulty occupational postures, general conditioning, and psychologic evaluation and intervention when indicated.

Temporomandibular Pain and Dysfunction Syndrome

Temporomandibular Pain and Dysfunction Syndrome, originally termed Costen's syndrome when described by Costen, is an arthralgia of the temporomandibular joint (TMJ). There are numerous theories, many concerning a dental malocclusion, but all also allude to the associated factors of musculoskeletal tension factors and posture. This latter aspect needs mention in any dissertation on neck and arm pain.

Pain is felt in the TMJ region slightly ahead of the ear and is associated with uncomfortable and even painful symptoms upon mastication: opening, biting, grinding, and lateral rotatory movements of the jaw. The patient may exhibit bruxism. This is usually nocturnal, but it can occasionally be diurnal. There is a clicking of the jaw upon opening.

Treatment of TMPDS includes dental occlusion evaluation and correction. An interarticular surgical procedure may be necessary if the meniscus(i) is damaged and occluding the joint motion. All methods of relaxation—such as biofeedback, operant conditioning, self-hypnosis, meditation—as well as postural and conditioning therapy should be employed.

PERICAPSULITIS SHOULDER PAIN

Because shoulder pain may be a referred pain from the cervical spine, the mere presence of shoulder pain prevents a differential diagnosis to be considered.

Shoulder pain and impairment usually has a mechanical basis of capsulitis from an inflamed supraspinatus tendon. The functional anatomy of the shoulder (Fig. 10–14) reveals that the major pathologic lesion is an *impingement tendonitis* of the supraspinatus tendon (Fig. 10–15). This may occur from abuse, such as excessive overhead motions, or from direct trauma, such as a fall on the outstretched arm. The history delineates the injury, and the examination reveals the tissue site of injury and the resultant impairment.

Supraspinatus tendonitis causes limited painful abduction of the arm at the glenohumeral joint (Fig. 10–16). In the attempt to abduct the arm, the failure of motion at this joint causes the scapulohumeral rhythm to be excessive in the

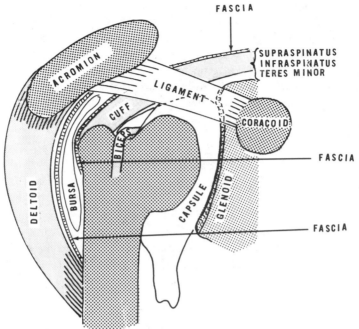

Figure 10–14. Tissue relationship of glenohumeral joint.

scapular phase; the shoulder shrugs instead of the arm abducting (Cailliet, 1981).

Rotator cuff tear may be complete or partial. In a complete tear the cuff tendon is disconnected from the greater tuberosity and thus can no longer externally rotate the head of the humerus. Abduction and active external rotation are no longer possible. Any attempt at abduction of the arm again is done with scapular motion alone.

In a partial rotator cuff tear, if enough cuff fibers remain intact, some—albeit weakened—abduction remains, but, because the remnants of the torn fibers bunch up, the painful reaction is the same as that in tendonitis: shrugging and pain at the painful arc site of abduction.

The pain in the shoulder region can thus be confirmed as coming from the cuff tendon pathology and not as a referred pain from cervical spine pathology. From chronic shrugging as a result of glenohumeral pathology, the scapular muscles that shrug the shoulder—the upper trapezius and the intercapular muscles—may cause pain in the neck as well as in the interscapular region. A careful examination delineates which component of shoulder pain is responsible.

The rounded upper back of faulty forward-head posture contributes to the occurrence of supraspinatus tendonitis and cervical diskogenic pain. In older people or in poorly postured, tense people with aggravating daily activities, both

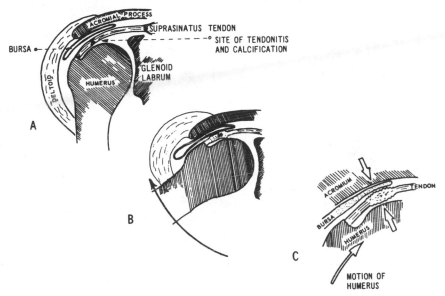

Figure 10–15. Glenohumeral movement. *(A)* Normal relationship of the humerus in the glenoid fossa under the overhang of the acromial process. The supraspinatus tendon runs in this groove and is protected by the subacromial, subdeltoid bursa. In normal movement, the humeral head depresses as it abducts and the tendon and the bursa move freely. *(B* and C) The tendon is frayed, inflamed, or even calcified; thus it is pinched between the humerus and the acromial process in arm abduction. Acute tendonitis and secondary bursitis result.

cervical radiculitis and shoulder peritendonitis may coexist. Both need evaluation and appropriate therapy. The shoulder's differential diagnosis is covered here, but not the therapy of shoulder pathology.

CARPAL TUNNEL SYNDROME

Pain or paresthesia felt in the hand occurring from median nerve compression at the wrist most frequently mimic the paresthesia referred from the cervical spine. The differentiation of median nerve wrist compression from cervical radiculitis or neurovascular bundle compression (TOS) may be the most challenging in clinical practice. Both may occur simultaneously, which further compounds the difficulty of precise diagnosis and appropriate treatment.

The cardinal symptoms of *carpal tunnel syndrome,* median nerve compression, are paresthesia and pain referred to the fingers and hand in the distribution of the median nerve (Fig. 10–17). Numbness of the fingers, muscular weakness, clumsiness, and possibly ultimate trophic changes noted in the finger are the

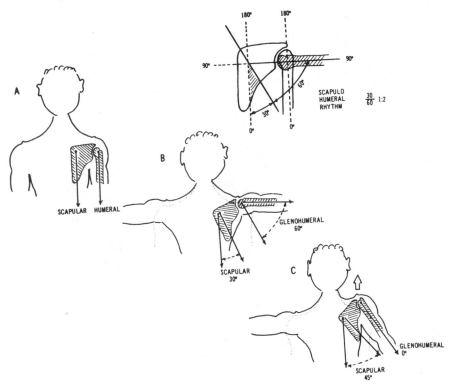

Figure 10–16. Scapulohumeral rhythm of shoulder movement. (A) Loose-hanging arm with the scapula and humerus at 0°. (B) Normal abduction during which, for every 15° of total abduction, 10° occur at the glenohumeral joint and 5° occur due to rotation of the scapula. (C) When obstruction exists at the glenohumeral joint, the scapular movement exceeds or is the only movement of the shoulder girdle, and *shrugging* occurs.

classic findings. The paresthesia is essentially numbness and tingling, termed *pins and needles,* that awaken the patient during the night or in early morning hours. The pain may have a burning quality, and the patient may qualify the clumsiness as "dropping things."

The objective verification of the hypalgesia or hypesthesia is loss of light touch and pin prick in the thumb and first two fingers—the median nerve distribution. The third and little finger sensation is usually spared, because this area is the dermatomal region of the ulnar nerve. There may be noted an elicited weakness in the median nerve myotomes: the abductor pollices and opponens pollices. In prolonged cases of entrapment, atrophy of the thenar eminence can be noted.

One manner of diagnosis is the Phalen test, which requires the reproduction of the median nerve paresthesia by forcefully flexing the wrist and holding

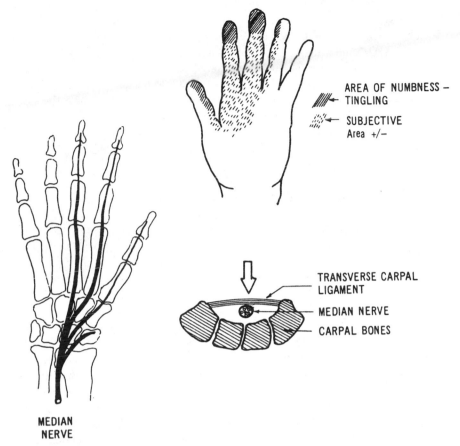

AREA OF NUMBNESS –
TINGLING

SUBJECTIVE
Area +/–

TRANSVERSE CARPAL
LIGAMENT

MEDIAN NERVE

CARPAL BONES

MEDIAN
NERVE

Figure 10–17. Carpal tunnel syndrome. Paresthesia and anesthesia occur from compression of the median nerve or its circulation at the carpal row of bone distal to the wrist. The compression occurs between the carpal bones and the transverse carpal ligament. The senior distribution is depicted. Of clinical significance is the absence of subjective and objective dysesthesia of the little finger. Compression of the compartment is clinically duplicated by a sustained flexion of the hand upon the forearm.

it in that position. In view of the fact that it is believed that the avascularity of the median nerve within the carpal tunnel causes the symptoms, application of a blood pressure cuff on the forearm and elevation of the pressure above arterial pressure for a period of time may reproduce the symptoms.

Direct digital percussion over the median nerve at the palmar area may elicit a positive Tinel sign, that is, a tingling in the median nerve distribution in an inflamed nerve. Relief of symptoms by use of a cock-up splint or an anesthetic steroid injection into the carpal tunnel is not only therapeutic but also diagnostic. These diagnostic tests differentiate the digital paresthesia from cervical radiculopathy or median nerve compression at the carpal tunnel.

Objective confirmation of carpal tunnel median nerve compression is possible with EMG and nerve conduction velocity studies. In cervical root entrapment a nerve conduction velocity would be normal, but the EMG could reveal similar irritation or demyelination studies of the C_5 to C_6 dermatomes and myotomes. A qualified electromyographer's evaluation is mandatory, as is the timing of the studies. Early findings may be normal but may change after a period of entrapment. Treatment should be employed for both conditions—the cervical spine and the wrist—while waiting for results of EMG studies.

BRACHIAL PLEXUS NEURITIS

This relatively infrequent neuritis should always be ruled out in upper extremity paresthesia and weakness if there is associated dermatomal pain. The onset is acute and usually consists of excruciating pain in the shoulder and down the arm. Weakness of the hand and arm is early and frequent and involves all the peripheral nerves of the upper extremities. Numbness of many dermatomes is noted early.

Diagnosis is difficult unless this neuritis occurs after a series of serum injections or a severe viral disease. Usually the etiology is unknown. Tests of inflammatory disease are of limited value, and early EMG studies are not indicative. The diagnosis is clinical by its subjective severity and the involvement of *all* nerve roots of the plexus.

Treatment is supportive to relieve pain. Local ice applications, immobilization with a sling, or elevation to afford relief is indicated. Oral or intramuscular medication may be needed during the early acute phase. Transcutaneous nerve stimulation or a stellate nerve block may be of value. Rehabilitation therapy is necessary to overcome the residual paresis or chronic pain that may result.

SHOULDER-HAND-FINGER SYNDROME

This example of reflex sympathetic dystrophy (RSD) should not be confused with cervical radiculopathy, but because there are similar symptoms and findings, it merits mention.

In shoulder-hand-finger syndrome the motion-limited, frequently painful shoulder is accompanied by pain, swelling, coldness, sweating, and color changes in the hand. A burning quality is usually associated with the pain in the hand.

There are often stages of RSD. First there is subjective burning, coldness, and a bluish appearance in a moist swollen hand. The skin is smooth, pale, and exquisitely tender to touch, air, or pressure. This stage may proceed to one of weakness, firmness of swelling, atrophy, and limited articular range of motion of the digits. The condition may ultimately progress to the more severe stage of severe atrophy, weakness, and stiffness, albeit painlessness.

Early treatment is mandatory to prevent progression of the hand to a useless appendage with chronic severe pain. Its relation to cervical radiculitis is apparent from the severity, the rapid and characteristic hand changes, and the diffuse distribution to more than one myotome and dermatome plus the ubiquitous stiff limited shoulder motion.

SUMMARY

Because many conditions may mimic the symptoms of cervical radiculopathy in the upper extremity, both locally and distally, it is mandatory that a precise differential diagnosis be established to ascertain appropriate treatment.

A full knowledge that these conditions may be present as causative of similar symptoms or in addition to the cervical radiculopathy is the beginning of proper diagnosis. Thorough knowledge of functional anatomy and the ability to elicit most symptoms with careful history and physical examination maneuvers is the prerequisite to correct diagnosis.

Understanding the pathomechanics as well as the tissue site of local and referred nociception leads to correct care of the impaired patient.

BIBLIOGRAPHY

Berg, PV: Myofascial pain syndromes. Postgrad Med 53:161, 1973.

Bonica, JJ: Management of myofascial pain syndrome in general practice. JAMA 133:732, 1957.

Buckelew, SP: Fibromyalgia: A rehabilitation approach. A Review. Am J Phys Med Rehabil 68(1):37, 1989.

Cailliet, R: Shoulder Pain, ed 2. FA Davis, Philadelphia, 1981.

Cailliet, R: Soft Tissue Pain and Disability, ed 2. FA Davis, Philadelphia, 1988.

Cloward, RB: Cervical diskography: A contribution to the etiology and mechanism of neck, shoulder, and arm pain. Ann Surg 150:229, 1947.

Costen, JB: A syndrome of ear and sinus problems dependent on disturbed function of the temporomandibular joint. Ann Otol Rhinol Laryngol 43:1, 1934.

Forster, FM and Kiesel, JA: Brachial plexus neuritis. Bulletin of Georgetown University Medical Center 5:74, 1951.

Gage, M and Parnell, H: Scalene anticus syndrome. Am J Surg 73:252, 1947.

Graham, W and Rosen, P: The shoulder-hand syndrome. Bull Rheum Dis 12:227, 1962.

Gunn, CC and Millbrandt, WE: Tenderness at motor points and aid in the diagnosis of pain in the shoulder referred from the cervical spine. JAOA 77:196, 1977.

Hall, CD: Clinical Concepts in Regional Musculoskeletal Illness. Grune & Stratton, London, 1987, p 227–244.

Johnson, EW, Wells, RM, and Duran, RJ: Diagnosis of carpal tunnel syndrome. Arch Phys Med Rehabil 43:414, 1962.

Kraft, GH, Johnson, EW, and LeBan, MM: The fibrositis syndrome. Arch Phys Med Rehabil 49:155, 1968.

Kraus, H: Use of surface anesthesia in treatment of painful motion. JAMA 116:2582, 1941

Kraus, H: Trigger points. NY State J Med 73:131, 1973.

McCain, GA and Scudds, RA: A review article: The concepts of primary fibromyalgia (fibrositis)—clinical value, relation and significance to other chronic musculoskeletal pain syndromes. Pain 33:273, 1988.

Michele, AA, et al: Scapulocostal syndrome (fatigue-postural paradox). NY State J Med 50:1353, 1950.

Molberg, E: Shoulder-hand-finger syndrome. Surg Clin North Am 40:367, 1948.

Moldofsky, H and Lue, FA: The relationship of alpha and delta EEG frequencies to pain and mood in "fibrositis" patients treated with chlorpromazine and L-tryptophane. Electroencephalogy Clin Neurophysiol 50:71, 1980.

Moldofsky, H, et al: Musculoskeletal symptoms and non-REM sleep disturbance in patients with "fibrositic syndrome" and healthy subjects. Psychosom Med 37:341, 1975.

Nachlas, IW: Scalenus anticus syndrome or cervical foraminal compression. South Med J 35:663, 1942.

Roos, DB: The thoracic outlet is underrated. Arch Neurol 47:327, 1990.

Simons, DG: Special review, muscle pain syndromes, Part II. Am J Phys Med 55:15, 1975.

Smythe, HA: "Fibrositis" as a disorder of pain modulation. Clin Rheum Dis 5:823, 1979.

Smythe, HA and Moldofsky, H: Two contributions to the understanding of the "fibrositis" syndrome. Bull Rheum Dis 28:928, 1977–1978.

Sola, AE and Kuitert, H: Myofascial trigger point pain in the neck and shoulder girdle: 100 cases treated by normal saline. Northwest Medicine 54:980, 1955.

Tegner, W, O'Neill, D, and Kaldegg, A: Psychogenic rheumatism. Br Med J 2:201, 1949.

Thorburn, W: The seventh cervical rib and its effect upon the brachial plexus. Medico-Chirugical Transactions 88:109, 1905.

Travell, JG and Simons, DG: Myofascial Pain and Dysfunction: The Trigger Point Manual. Williams & Wilkins, Baltimore, 1983.

Tsairis, P, Dyke, PJ, and Mulder, DW: Natural history of brachial plexus neuropathy. Arch Neurol 27:109, 1972.

Tyson, RR and Kaplan, GF: Modern concepts of diagnosis and treatment of the thoracic outlet syndrome. Orthop Clin North Am 6(2):507, 1975.

Urschel, HC, et al: Objective diagnosis (ulnar nerve conduction velocity) and current therapy of the thoracic outlet syndrome. Ann Thorac Surg 12:608, 1971.

Urschel, HG, et al: Objective diagnosis (ulnar nerve conduction velocity) and current therapy of the thoracic outlet syndrome. Ann Thorac Surg 12 (6):603, 1971.

Wilbourn, AJ: The thoracic outlet syndrome is overdiagnosed. Arch Neurol 47:328, 1990.

Woods, WW: Personal experience with surgical treatment of 250 cases of cervicobrachial neurovascular compression syndrome. Journal of the International College of Surgeons 44(3):273, 1965.

Yunus, M, Masi, AT, and Aldag, JC: Criteria studies of primary fibromyalgia syndrome (PFS) (abstr). Arthritis and Rheumatism 30:27C, 1987.

INDEX

An "f" following a page number indicates a figure.